W9-BHT-386

Study Guide
for

Pharmacology and the Nursing Process
Third Edition

Linda Lane Lilley, PhD, RN
Robert S. Aucker, PharmD

Julie S. Snyder, MSN, RN, C
Faculty, School of Nursing
Louise Obici Memorial Hospital
Suffolk, Virginia

with special thanks to
Linda K. Wendling
for her contribution to the first edition

Study Skills by
Richard E. Lake, BS, MS, MLA
Director, Center for Student Success
Professor, Reading Department
St. Louis Community College at Florissant Valley
St. Louis, Missouri

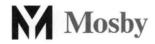 Mosby

A Harcourt Health Sciences Company

St. Louis   London   Philadelphia   Sydney   Toronto

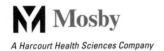

Vice President and Publishing Director: Sally Schrefer
Executive Editor: Robin Carter
Senior Developmental Editor: Kristin Geen
Project Manager: Gayle Morris
Production Editor: Stephanie Hebenstreit
Designer: Amy Buxton

THIRD EDITION
Copyright © 2002 by Mosby, Inc.

Previous editions copyrighted 1996, 1999.

All rights reserved. No part of this publication may be reproduced or transmitted in any form or by any means, electronic or mechanical, including photocopy, recording, or any information storage and retrieval system, without permission in writing from the publisher.

Permission to photocopy or reproduce solely for internal or personal use is permitted for libraries or other users registered with the Copyright Clearance Center, provided that the base fee of $4.00 per chapter plus $.10 per page is paid directly to the Copyright Clearance Center, Inc., 222 Rosewood Drive, Danvers, MA 01923. This consent does not extend to other kinds of copying, such as copying for general distribution, for advertising or promotional purposes, for creating new collected works, or for resale.

Mosby, Inc.
A Harcourt Health Sciences Company
11830 Westline Industrial Drive
St. Louis, Missouri 63146

Printed in the United States of America

Composition by Wordbench

International Standard Book Number: 0-323-01269-8

01 02 03 04 05 WB/EB 9 8 7 6 5 4 3 2 1

Table of Contents

Overview of Dosage Calculations

Answers

Student Study Tips

TIME MANAGEMENT

If there is one consistent cry from college students, it is: "I don't have enough time." The quantity of work to be done always seems to exceed the time available for completing it. There is thus no skill that can do more to reduce anxiety and increase effectiveness than learning to manage your time effectively.

Although it is not possible to control your time, it is possible to manage certain portions of it. This is an important distinction. *Control* implies complete power over time, but this is simply not true. Life is filled with unexpected surprises that make control of time impossible. A sick child, a traffic jam, a schedule change at work—the list of possible surprises is nearly endless. Those who set out to control time are doomed to fail. However, each of us can learn to manage time, to use the time we have available more productively.

General Guidelines

Some tasks are best accomplished using schedules and lists; others are more easily accomplished by specifying goals coupled with the steps to be taken to achieve these goals. Regardless of the specific tools used to manage time, there are three important factors to be considered. First, there are only 24 hours in a day, and there is absolutely nothing we can do to increase this number. Second, we generally underestimate the time it will take to complete a given task. Therefore, as a general guideline, it is best to double the estimated time for completion. This should always allow sufficient time for completing the job. If the task takes less time than that allocated, the remaining time can be used either for other tasks or for doing something recreational as a reward for a job well done. Third, there are only two ways you can find more time to do the things you need to do: either do the job faster or learn to use your time more effectively. Doing the job faster is not really a very successful approach because the faster you try to get things done, the more likely you are to make mistakes, which only have to be corrected later, and this costs time in the long run. Studying a complex and technical subject such as pharmacology cannot be done rapidly—not if you want to understand and remember what you have studied. This means the only real solution to increasing the time you have is to manage your time more successfully. This takes skill, and like all skills, it can be learned. Everyone can learn to be more effective, but you must approach the learning of this skill with a positive attitude. Remember this is the tool that gets you started. It is easy to procrastinate, but procrastination is like nailing the toe of one shoe to the floor before you put it on—there is lots of motion but no progress. Knowing how to use your time effectively is the way to *get started*.

Tasks to Be Managed

There are three kinds of tasks. There are those jobs that *have to be done,* such things as going to class, going to work, eating, and getting adequate rest. These jobs are the easiest to accomplish because the consequences of not doing them are serious. If you don't go to class, failure is almost a sure thing. If you don't go to work, soon there will be no paycheck. The consequences of not eating or sleeping are obvious. The "have to" jobs don't require much in the way of time management, because these tasks are usually scheduled by others anyway.

The second kind of task is the job that *should be done.* This includes things such as studying, paying bills, cleaning house, and all those other necessary but unpleasant tasks that are part of life. The "should be done" jobs are the most difficult of the three kinds to accomplish because they are the jobs that are all too easy to put off doing. These are also the jobs where time management skills are most essential.

The third kind of task is the one we *want to do.* These "tasks" encompass all the fun things that provide pleasure and escape from the routines of class, study, and work, but they are also all too easy to find time for. In fact most of us are very successful at finding time to do what we want to do, even when there is a sizable backlog of "should-be-done"

Copyright © 2002 by Mosby, Inc. All rights reserved.

chores waiting. This third category of tasks should not be overlooked when it comes to managing time because they can serve as the stimulus to getting started on "should-be-done" tasks, and as the reward for getting them done. Some recreation time is absolutely essential in any effective time management system.

Rewards

As just mentioned, recreation time can be a highly effective incentive for getting required tasks done. It serves as the gold stars and M&Ms you may have had teachers give you in grade school as a reward for a job well done. Students in grade school will often work very hard at tasks set by the teacher in order to earn a gold star on a paper or a handful of M&Ms. Although such rewards can motivate grade school students, in nursing programs M&Ms and gold stars are pretty much a thing of the past. Besides this, such rewards lose some of their value as we grow up, though the concept of reward is still important. You need a new kind of gold star to help motivate you. For each person the rewards may be very different, and you may have to spend a little time determining what will work for you. It might be watching your favorite soap opera, a prime time drama, or comedy show; going to the movie theater to see a new release; reading a book for pleasure; or it might just be spending some time with family or friends.

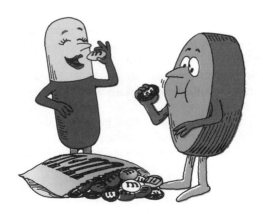

Types of Schedules
Master Schedule: An Essential First Step

The first step in effectively managing your time is to create a 7-day worksheet. To do this, draw seven columns, each one representing one day of the week, beginning with Sunday in column 1 and ending with Saturday in column 7. Then divide each column into blocks representing 1 hour of time each. Start at the top of the page with the time you usually get up in the morning and end each column with the time when you usually go to bed. A typical master schedule might begin at 6 A.M. and end at 11 P.M. Once the blank sheet is prepared, the next step is to fill in those hours that are already scheduled. These are the hours others control, and the activities are those that occur at the same hour, on the same day or days, and for several weeks or longer. For example, the semester's schedule of classes is the first activity to enter into a master schedule. Other activities such as work, travel, worship services, and any other regular activities also belong in the master schedule. The master schedule should consist only of those recurring activities that cannot be done at any other time. Activities such as doing the laundry, watching television, and shopping should not be included because the time when you do them is more flexible. The idea behind the master schedule is to establish those times of the day that are "spent" and therefore cannot be used for any other activities. The empty blocks that remain represent the time you have to do everything else. Fig. 1-1 shows a sample master schedule.

The master schedule is an essential first step in managing time effectively. Whether you think of schedules as too restrictive or enjoy the feeling of control that a good schedule affords, it is still necessary to prepare a master schedule. This schedule tells you when you have time to complete the "should-be-done" and "want-to-do" tasks. Creating a master schedule takes no more than a half hour, but it will generally serve you for an entire semester. The only reason for doing a new master schedule is when some significant schedule change occurs. For instance, if you get a new work assignment or your nursing practicum site changes and requires an additional 15 or 20 minutes of travel time each way, then a new master schedule should be drawn up to accommodate the increase or decrease in time that is now required. Once the master schedule is done, make four or five copies of it. These copies will be used to prepare the detailed weekly schedule.

Detailed Weekly Schedule

The detailed weekly schedule is more complex. It is intended to help you plan for study, recreation, family, and all those other activities that need to be fitted into a typical week. To make out the detailed weekly schedule, take one of the copies you have made of the master schedule and begin to fill in the open blocks of time. The first blocks of time you should fill in are the most important ones for any

Copyright © 2002 by Mosby, Inc. All rights reserved.

MASTER SCHEDULE EXAMPLE

	SUN	MON	TUES	WED	THUR	FRI	SAT
7:00		GET UP		GET UP		GET UP	
8:00		TRAVEL		TRAVEL		TRAVEL	
9:00	GET UP	CLASS		CLASS		CLASS	
10:00	CHURCH	CLASS	TRAVEL	CLASS	TRAVEL	CLASS	
11:00	CHURCH		PRACTICUM		PRACTICUM		
12:00		CLASS	PRACTICUM	CLASS	PRACTICUM		
1:00			PRACTICUM		PRACTICUM		
2:00		PERSONAL	PRACTICUM		PRACTICUM		
3:00		PERSONAL					
4:00		AEROBICS		AEROBICS		AEROBICS	
5:00							
6:00		DINNER	DINNER	DINNER	DINNER	DINNER	
7:00							FUN
8:00							FUN
9:00							FUN
10:00							FUN
11:00	BEDTIME	BEDTIME	BEDTIME	BEDTIME	BEDTIME	BEDTIME	FUN

▼ **FIG. 1-1.** The master schedule. This is an essential first step in managing time effectively.

student—study time. This is what time management is all about—scheduling the needed hours of study (Fig. 1-2).

Before filling in any study hours, there are a number of important factors you must consider. First is the amount of planned study time. There is an old rule pertaining to study time, and even though it is an old rule, it is still a very good guideline. The rule is to plan 2 hours of study time for each 1 hour spent in class. For example, a 3-credit-hour course meets 3 hours per week, so you need to plan 6 hours of study time per week for this course. Remember, this is a general rule. Some courses will not actually require as much time as you allot, while others will require more. The reason for beginning a semester with this approach is simple. It is easy to find things to do with time you don't need for study, but once a semester is under way it can be very difficult to find additional study time. If you don't plan enough study time at the beginning, you will soon find yourself in a constant battle to keep up. This is followed by frustration, anxiety, and a sense of impending doom, feelings you don't need when you want to perform at your very best.

A second factor you must consider when making out a detailed weekly schedule is your personal "clock." Do you wake up early, ready to charge forward? Do you do your best work during the early hours of the day but find it very difficult to be productive after 10 P.M.? Or do you wake up early only because a certain course meets at 8 A.M. and you have to be there? Do you do your best work in the afternoon and early evening and prefer to sleep until 10 A.M.? Are you a night owl? These are questions you must answer when scheduling study time. You are determining your prime time, those times of the day when your ability to concentrate is at its best and you can accomplish the most. These are the times you want to use for study whenever possible. It is not usually possible, because of class and work schedules, to schedule all study time in your prime hours, but it is essential that those hours be used for study as much as possible. It would be foolish to plan to study your toughest material between 9 and 11 P.M., when you know that is a time when just reading the daily paper is a challenge.

The third aspect to preparing a detailed schedule is to allot some study hours for specific courses and some simply as study hours. The reason for doing this is that the study demands of courses vary from day to day and week to week. For instance, you will need some hours of study every week to master new material, terms, and concepts in pharmacology, but the study time demands will increase in the days just before exams, midterms, and project due dates. The hours set aside for specific courses

Copyright © 2002 by Mosby, Inc. All rights reserved.

DETAILED WEEKLY SCHEDULE EXAMPLE

	SUN	MON	TUES	WED	THUR	FRI	SAT
7:00		GET UP		GET UP		GET UP	
8:00		TRAVEL		TRAVEL		TRAVEL	
9:00	GET UP	CLASS	STUDY	CLASS	STUDY	CLASS	
10:00	CHURCH	CLASS	TRAVEL	CLASS	TRAVEL	CLASS	STUDY
11:00	CHURCH	LUNCH	PRACTICUM	LUNCH	PRACTICUM	LUNCH	STUDY
12:00		CLASS	PRACTICUM	CLASS	PRACTICUM		PERSONAL
1:00		STUDY	PRACTICUM	STUDY	PRACTICUM	STUDY	PERSONAL
2:00	FREE	STUDY	PRACTICUM	STUDY	PRACTICUM	STUDY	PERSONAL
3:00			TRAVEL		TRAVEL		
4:00		AEROBICS		AEROBICS		AEROBICS	
5:00							
6:00		DINNER	DINNER	DINNER	DINNER	DINNER	
7:00	STUDY	STUDY	STUDY	STUDY	STUDY	STUDY	FUN
8:00	STUDY		STUDY		STUDY		FUN
9:00	STUDY	REVIEW	REVIEW	REVIEW	REVIEW		FUN
10:00							FUN
11:00	BEDTIME	BEDTIME	BEDTIME	BEDTIME	BEDTIME	BEDTIME	FUN

▼ **FIG. 1-2.** The detailed weekly schedule. Fill in the study times first.

are for accomplishing the day-to-day study demands; the unassigned study hours are for meeting the changing demands posed by these special circumstances. These unassigned study hours also let you meet unexpected demands. No matter how carefully you plan your time, it is a certainty that something will happen to prevent you from using the time block you had set aside for learning.

It usually takes two or three attempts over a period of 3 weeks or so to arrive at a detailed schedule that works well for you. There is a tendency on the first attempt to try to schedule some important activity for every waking hour. Ultimately (usually within a couple of days) this schedule will make you feel as though there is no time for anything but work. Don't let that discourage you from the idea of a schedule. Instead, evaluate what was working and what was not working in the old schedule, and then make a new detailed weekly schedule that takes your findings into account. This second schedule will come much closer to being realistic and effective. Sometimes this second attempt will yield a schedule that works fine for the balance of the semester. However, if this second effort doesn't quite "fill the bill," then evaluate it and prepare a third version. This third attempt will usually prove to be successful. The need to evaluate and revise is the reason for making several copies of the master schedule. It saves time in the revision process, and saving time is, after all, what time management is all about.

Daily Schedules and Lists

The final stage in time management is the daily schedule or "to do" list. No matter how carefully and thoughtfully a detailed weekly schedule is prepared, it simply cannot include all the tasks you will face. These consist of small tasks, infrequent tasks, and unexpected tasks. This is where the daily schedule comes in. Each day as you think of things you want or need to do the next day, write them down. Carry a small notebook that will fit into a pocket or purse or, my personal preference, a packet of 3 × 5 note cards for jotting these items down. Each night, just before bedtime, review the list for the next day.

Daily Priorities

Set priorities. Many people make up daily lists and then become frustrated because they can't accomplish all the jobs on the list. Usually this is the result of listing everything they think of without any thought to the relative importance of the task.

Copyright © 2002 by Mosby, Inc. All rights reserved.

For example, going to the dry cleaners is critical if the outfit you must wear tomorrow is there. But if you don't absolutely have to have that outfit tomorrow, then the trip to the cleaners is a very low priority and can be postponed to another day. Yes, this is a form of procrastination, and procrastination is the worst enemy of time management, but at the same time, the object of time management is to get the job done when it must be done. If the job doesn't have to be done immediately and the day is going to be a full one, then postponing unimportant tasks is actually good management.

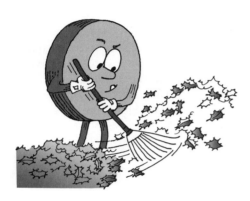

Look carefully at the list and number the tasks according to their importance; this sets the priority and really makes the day productive.

There are some helpful rules to apply when setting priorities. First, be realistic. Don't put items on the list that can't possibly be done on that day. Don't plan to review three chapters of text material on a day when you know there will not be enough time to cover more than half of one chapter. Second, apply the 80/20 rule, which states that 80% of what you must do will probably constitute 20% of the list. If your daily list consists of ten items, it is likely that two or at most three of them will consume 80% of your time and be the most important ones on the list. Applying the 80/20 rule really helps establish personal priorities. Finally, look at the small tasks listed, tasks such as picking up milk and dog food, dropping off dry cleaning, and going to the bank. Plan not only to do those errands but also think about the order in which they should be done. If you can plan your route so that it completes a circle from home to cleaners to grocery to home, it will be much more time efficient than going from home to grocery, back home, then to the cleaner, and finally back home again.

As you complete a job on the daily list, cross it off—big and bold. Crossing it off tells you that you are making progress and at the same time motivates you to move to the next item on the list. At the end of the day there is no feeling quite so satisfying as looking at the daily list and finding every item crossed off (and sometimes even one or two last-minute additions as well). If not every item is crossed off, don't look on the day as a failure. Remember the 80/20 rule. If you accomplished 80% of the tasks on the list, it was a productive day. Daily lists can really help you get the job done.

Goals and Actions

Schedules and lists work well for accomplishing most tasks but can fail in certain situations. Complex tasks that take several days to complete or that extend over a period of several weeks often don't fit neatly into a schedule. There is another simple way to manage time that works really well in these situations. It involves establishing a goal and then a plan of action to reach the goal.

Guidelines for Setting Goals

There are some basic guidelines to be followed in setting goals.

- **Be realistic.**
  The goal must be something that you can reasonably expect to accomplish. A goal of 100% on each and every unit test is not realistic. A goal of 85% or better is.
- **Be specific.**
  Goals must set out exactly what it is that needs to be done. Don't simply state "I will study for the exam." Specify how many hours, what days, and what times you will study. The more specific the goal statement, the easier it is to establish a plan, complete that plan, and thus achieve the goal set.
- **Set a time limit.**
  Specify a time limit for completing each step in the plan and an overall deadline for completing the goal.
- **Make goal and actions measurable.**
  State the goal and each step in the plan for achieving it in a way that will enable you to measure your progress toward completion.

Following is an example of how this goal and action process works: You have a chapter test a week from today. The test will cover approximately 45 pages of text material, and there are 40 specific pharmacologic terms you must know. In addition, you have been given about 20 pages of supplementary handouts in class. What will you do in the next seven days to prepare for this test?

Copyright © 2002 by Mosby, Inc. All rights reserved.

Goal statement

I will study to make a good grade on this exam.

This is a poor goal statement because it is not specific, sets no time limits, and offers no real way to measure progress. The intent is good, but the implementation of such a vague goal is usually poor.

Revision 1

I will spend 2 hours a day studying for the next chapter test in order to get at least an 80% score.

This is a better goal statement. Assuming the 2 hours per day is realistic, the goal is more specific, the grade goal is measurable, and there is a sort of time limit. This goal statement might be good enough, but it could still be improved.

Final version

I will spend 2 hours per day, from 2:30 to 4:30 P.M., for the next 7 days studying for the chapter test in order to score at least 80%.

This is what is needed. It states how much time, when, how many days, and the purpose. Setting clear goals helps you get started and serves as a motivator to keep you working.

Guidelines for Action Statements

A goal, no matter how well stated, is not enough. There must be action statements to help you make day-to-day progress toward meeting the goal. The guidelines that apply to defining your goal also apply to the action statements: they should be realistic, specific, measurable, and time-limited. Action statements are much like the "to do" lists discussed under time management. They spell out what is going to be done day to day. Here are three examples of good action statements for the sample goal.

■ I will master six pharmacology terms each day.
■ I will spend from 2:30 to 3:00 P.M. each day reviewing class handouts.
■ I will review 10 pages of text material from 3:00 to 4:00 P.M. each day.

These statements should give you a good idea of how to go about developing a clear goal and a set of actions to carry out to achieve that goal. Using the scheduling techniques and the goal-and-actions process will make you a highly effective time manager and a very productive student. The detailed weekly schedule comes into play when you are doing an action plan. Look at it to find the days and times to set aside for accomplishing the steps in your plan.

On-the-Run Study

There are many study activities that can be accomplished in relatively small blocks of time of 5, 10, or 15 minutes. Small blocks of time are often lost or wasted because it doesn't seem as though anything significant could be accomplished in them. If you learn to use them effectively, this can free up larger blocks for more time-consuming tasks. If a class ends 10 minutes early, use the time for study. If you are waiting for your ride, use the time for study. Take advantage of such "found" time to review five vocabulary terms, rework a set of class notes, or preview the next 5 pages of assigned reading. Studying on the run may free up an hour or more for concentrated study or for recreation. Every free minute does not have to be devoted to study; recreation time (camp counselors call it "me time") is important, too. But using the odd minutes in the day to advantage can really help you achieve your goals as a student. Watch throughout this chapter for specific activities that can be done on the run.

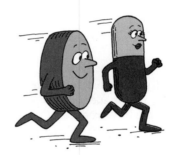

NOTE-TAKING—LECTURES

Taking quality lecture notes is not easy. Most of us have never been taught how to take notes, yet note-taking is a complex and important process. Even more important than the notes you take, however, is what you do with them after class. No matter how good or how poor your class notes are, they are of limited use if they are not used effectively. Too often notes taken during a lecture are ignored until a day or two before the exam, at which time the student discovers that some of the notes are unclear, unreadable, or even useless.

Why Take Notes?

The primary reason for taking notes is obvious. It is impossible to remember everything that is said during a 1- to 2-hour lecture period, so we take notes as an aid to memory for review at a later time. Second, the act of writing something down helps to strengthen learning and memory. Finally, note-

Copyright © 2002 by Mosby, Inc. All rights reserved.

taking helps us to focus our attention on the lecture. It is very easy to drift off into the land of daydreams during a lecture; note-taking helps keep us involved.

Note-Taking Problems

The biggest single problem for every note-taker is selectivity—deciding what must be in the notes. It is impossible and unnecessary to write down every word the lecturer says. But it is critically important that concepts, terms, and useful examples are noted. There is also the problem of unfamiliar vocabulary, which is even more noticeable in a course heavy on technical, medical, and pharmaceutical terminology such as this one. Yet another problem for some is the simple matter of hard-to-read or even illegible handwriting. Finally, there is the problem of trying to listen and write at the same time. All of these problems can make note-taking very difficult. But it is also important to understand that note-takers are made, not born. You can learn to be more effective as both a note-taker and note-user, but it requires some practice and a willingness to adopt new techniques.

How to Take Notes

Note-taking is much more than simply jotting some words down on paper during a lecture, then not looking at these notes again until some later date—often the night before the test. Note-taking is a multiple-stage process that is spread out over the days and weeks between the lecture and the time when you are reviewing your notes in preparation for a test. There are five stages in the note-taking process, which, if followed, will make you a better note-taker and a more successful student.

Stage One—Prereading
Stage Two—Listening and Observation
Stage Three—In-Class Note-Taking
Stage Four—Out-of-Class Rework
Stage Five—Frequent, Active Review

Stage One—Prereading

Note-taking begins before the lecture. Taking quality notes during a lecture is never easy, but going into class unprepared for the lecture compounds the problem. Read any and all assigned material before class. This provides you with the background needed to listen intelligently to the lecture and to be selective when taking notes. If you go into a lecture without reading the related material, you may find that it is like listening to a foreign language, with only bits and pieces making any

sense. One reason for this is that the vocabulary will be unfamiliar. Without the background gained from reading the assigned material, it will be very difficult to get down the important ideas, terms, and facts. Without this background understanding, everything said will seem important, with the result that you end up with notes that aren't really very helpful when it comes time to review them in preparation for an exam.

Stage Two—Listening and Observation

Taking quality class notes requires active listening. This is one of the most challenging aspects of being a good note-taker. It requires an awareness of both the lecturer's language and his or her nonverbal style. You have to pay attention not only to what is said, the verbal aspect, but also to the visual, nonverbal, aspect of the presentation.

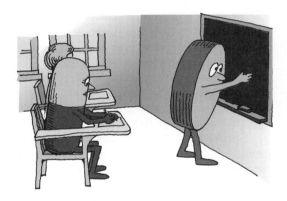

As already stressed, it is not necessary to write down everything that is said. The objective is to be selective, focusing on the most important ideas, terms, and facts to be recorded for later review. If you spend the lecture time trying to write down every word, you will not be able to listen to and therefore grasp the ideas. Writing less and listening more is a good rule to follow for note-taking.

Learn to listen for key words and phrases. What are these key words and phrases? They vary with the subject content and with the individual lecturer, so there is no way to provide a single, definitive list of them. However, there are some verbal signals (words) that will give you clues to important information the lecturer is about to give.

Sequence words—"first," "second," "next," "then," "last," "finally"
Contrast words—"but," "however," "on the other hand"

Copyright © 2002 by Mosby, Inc. All rights reserved.

Importance words—"significant," "key," "main," "main point," "most important"

The use of words and phrases such as these is the lecturer's way of signaling the relative importance and progression of certain facts and ideas. Also remember that, as important as the words are, it is also necessary to be aware of the volume, tone, and pace of delivery. All of these factors combine to form the speaker's verbal style.

There is another aspect of the lecture that must also be considered—the nonverbal signals. Observe your instructor carefully. Watch his or her hand gestures, eye contact, classroom location, and overall body language. These nonverbal signals add emphasis to the lecture. If the instructor says, "One of the most important drugs in the treatment of . . ." this should immediately tell you that what follows is an important point for your notes. The instructor has even told you it is important. If, at the same time, the instructor looks directly at one student, moves nearer to the class, speaks more loudly, slowly, or rapidly, or makes an emphatic gesture, this also tells you that the particular piece of information that is to be given is almost certainly going to be included on the next test. As you practice listening and observing in the lecture environment, you will find that your ability to discern the important ideas grows.

Stages one and two are preparation for the real work that goes on in the last three stages.

Split-Page Note Format. The split-page format requires a change in the way you set up your notepaper. This involves dividing each sheet into two parts by drawing a line down the full length of the page, creating a left-hand column that is 2½ to 3 inches in width and a right-hand column that is 5½ to 6 inches in width. The right-hand column should be used for taking class notes. (The function of the left-hand column will be explained in the description of stages four and five.)

Stage Three—In-Class Note-Taking

There is no magic formula for note-taking. Simply take the best notes you possibly can. Remember, notes are personal. Don't judge your notes against those of other classmates. Some will take lots of notes, and others with a different background and expectations will take far fewer notes. However, there are some simple tips for taking notes that will make the process easier and also make for better notes.

Write in your own words most of the time. Writing ideas in your own style will make them easier to learn and remember.

Leave space between main points. When you sense that the lecturer has moved to a new idea, leave a couple of lines blank on your note paper. That way if the lecturer returns to this point later, you will have room to add further notes. Even if there is no need for additional notes, the blank lines will help you to see the organization of the ideas and the relationship between them.

Be aware of **direct cues** from the lecturer, such as "this will be on the test, "this is a difficult concept," or even "know this." Statements like these tell you something is important and will probably be on future tests.

Be especially aware of the **visual presentation.** This consists of information written on the chalkboard or displayed on an overhead projector, slide projector, or other electronic displays. Many lecturers outline key points on the chalkboard as a means of staying focused on the points they want to cover. Use this information to help you stay equally focused. Electronic displays are often chosen because the ideas can best be understood when presented visually.

The **repetition** of certain points is the single most useful tip that they are really important. When an idea, term, or fact is important, the lecturer will almost certainly repeat it. For instance, the lecturer will introduce a new term, define it, give a couple of examples to clarify the definition, and finally redefine the term. This repetition is a signal that it is very important for you to learn the information.

Another technique used by lecturers, which you can use as a note-taker, is **questions directed to the class.** These questions are another way the speaker stresses important information and are also a way for him or her to find out how well the students have understood what has been said. Such questions are thus also cues that certain information is important.

Don't simply sit, listen, and let words and sentences wash over you like waves on the beach. To take quality notes you have to be **actively involved** in what is going on in class. This means being willing to respond to a question directed to the class. It also means asking questions of the speaker when things are not clear. Don't feel that because no one else is asking questions you are the only person who doesn't understand something. It is highly probable that there are others who are just as confused. Your objective in class is to understand the lecture and record key ideas in your notes so that you can study effectively. Questions are *not dumb* if they relate to the material being presented.

Copyright © 2002 by Mosby, Inc. All rights reserved.

Stage Four—Out-of-Class Rework

The notes you take in class are only a part of the effective study of lecture material. The next stage, out-of-class reworking of these notes, is critical, and this is where the left-hand column of your notepaper comes into use. This reworking must take place on the same day as the lecture. Ideally it should be done immediately after the class ends, but this is not always possible. It must, however, be done that day, and the sooner the better. Reworking class notes won't take more than 10 to 15 minutes to complete, but it will save you hours of study time later on.

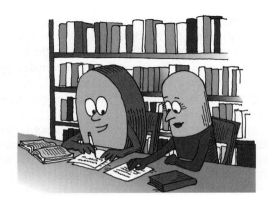

Following is the recommended method for reworking your class notes.

1. **Read over the class notes.** Read for the lecture's organization. At this point you are not trying to remember everything you got from the lecture but trying to see what the major topics and key ideas and terms are. You should also be looking for places where your notes are incomplete or confusing. If you read your notes soon after the lecture, you will be able to clarify points or add missing material because most of what was said will still be fresh in your mind. If you wait until the next day (or worse, the next week), what is now only confusing will by then be a complete mystery. Taking the time to read your notes over soon after you take them will save much time and frustration later on.

2. **Write topic heads for lecture segments.** As you read your notes, identify the major topics that were discussed. Look, for example, at Chapter 10 in the text. The chapter title tells you that it is about general and local anesthetics, but it doesn't stop there. "Stages of Anesthesia" is named as the topic, and this is further divided into "Induction," "Excitement," "Surgical," and so on. These headings are necessary to break down very complex material into understandable blocks. You should be doing the same thing with your notes. Write topic labels such as these in the left-hand column of your notes. Limit your labels to three to five words. You are not trying to rewrite class notes but to make the organization of the ideas crystal clear. Sometimes the notes on the chalkboard will provide the labels for you. Sometimes the labels will be included in a lesson outline furnished by the instructor. Often, however, you will have to compose your own labels. It is not easy at first to come up with these headings, but with practice you will develop the skill. Keep at it. These labels are an essential aspect of the final stage of this note-taking method.

3. **List vocabulary.** The left-hand column is also a great place to put content-specific vocabulary. Look again at Chapter 10. Notice that there is a glossary of terms for that chapter. This is provided so that you can immediately begin to focus on the content-specific vocabulary you will have to master for that chapter. You can create your own personal glossary of the terms used in lecture. As you read over your notes, each time you encounter terms from the text or new terms introduced in the lecture, note the word in the left-hand column. By doing this, you have set into motion the process for learning needed vocabulary.

4. **Expand.** Often during a lecture, you will only have time to write fragments of information. These may be meaningful at the time you write them but can later be very confusing. Therefore, as you read your notes, fill in those places where there may be such gaps; otherwise, what was a small problem will become a big one later on. It won't take long, and it will pay off. You may use the left-hand column for adding such information.

Remember: The reworking must be done the same day as the lecture for it to be efficient and productive. The longer the interval between the lecture and this reworking, the greater the likelihood for forgetting. When you read notes the same day as the lecture, you will be able to recall almost everything said. Wait until tomorrow, and . . . ! The reworking process will only take 10 minutes or so to complete, but it will pay off in a significantly improved set of class notes. Of equal importance is the fact that the reworking process is preparation for the final, critical stage in the note-taking process.

Stage Five—Frequent, Active Review

Notes, no matter how good, need to be studied early and often. Learning and memory depend on rehearsal, or review, and this must be an active

Copyright © 2002 by Mosby, Inc. All rights reserved.

process. Rereading notes will improve your understanding and memory somewhat, but there is a technique you can use that will accomplish much more. This technique will help you to be an active learner and encourage frequent rehearsal. It is also efficient because it will only take you 10 to 15 minutes to completely review 2 or 3 days' worth of class notes.

When to Review. The first review of your notes should be done within 2 days of the lecture. If the lecture has taken place on Monday, your review should occur on Tuesday or Wednesday. Don't wait more than 2 days. Studies have repeatedly shown that we forget nearly 50% of what we learn in the first 24 hours after we learn it. The reworking process will slow the forgetting process, but it will not stop it. The longer you wait to review your notes, the more time it will take and the more difficult it will be when you do.

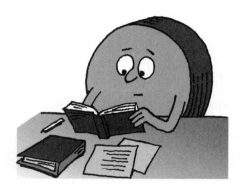

When to do a second, third, or any additional reviews depends on the success of the previous review. Review each day until you find that you remember and understand 80% or more of the material (you have to be the judge). When this is accomplished, the next review can wait for 3 or 4 days. If you find that after the first review you recall or understand only 70% of the material (an average amount), then the next review should occur within 2 or 3 days. If the amount you remember is less than 70%, you should review the material the next day. You must assess your own performance on each review to determine how soon to schedule another review. There are no hard-and-fast rules for this. A good review does not mean you have mastered the material forever, and what you clearly remember at one review may be the very thing you forget the next time around. **The only rule is to review frequently.** By doing this you will be well prepared for quizzes, tests, or any other measures of your learning.

How to Review. To review your notes, cover the right-hand column (class notes) with a blank sheet of paper. Look at the topics, vocabulary, and further notes that you added to the left-hand column during the reworking process. These will serve as your study guide for review. Look at the first topic heading you've written. It might be something like "Hypnotics" (Chapter 11). Turn that heading into one or more questions. *What are hypnotics? When are they used? What are the side effects? Are there persons for whom hypnotics are inappropriate?* Ask these questions *aloud;* don't just think them. Framing questions orally is what makes this review active. Now that you have asked a question, the next step is obvious. Answer it without looking at the covered notes. The answer should also be spoken aloud. This oral question-and-answer process forces you to state the information in your own words and style. In addition, you are relying on more faculties in your learning than just the visual aspect of rereading. You are speaking and listening, which is more active than just looking at the words. Recall is strongly enhanced by expressing the information in your own words.

Another benefit of this review process is that it helps identify what you don't know. If you ask a question and find yourself struggling to respond, then it should be clear that this is something you have not yet mastered. When this happens, uncover the class notes pertaining to that topic and read what is needed. Sometimes it will only require three or four words to trigger recall. When this happens, immediately cover the notes and resume your oral response. Sometimes it will require your reading a large portion of the notes to trigger your memory. What is important is that the reading is now focused on material that you have clearly identified as unknown. This means that your review time will be much more productive. Instead of reading everything known and unknown, you will now be concentrating on reinforcing the known material and studying the unknown. The best way to prepare for a test is to take a test. By using the question-and-answer model you are creating and taking your own test. You may discover that many of the questions you asked yourself also appear in some form on the classroom test covering that same material. If you have already answered the question several times for yourself, it will be very easy to answer it on the test.

Two-Page Split Note Variation. There is a variation of the split-page notepaper format that some students find works better for them. If you find that the 6-inch-wide right-hand column is too narrow for taking class notes, simply take your class

Copyright © 2002 by Mosby, Inc. All rights reserved.

notes on the right-hand page in your notebook and use the left-hand page for the reworking process. This allows more room for the charts, diagrams, or complex formulas that are often part of the lecture material in courses such as pharmacology. This two-page model will also allow you to incorporate text notes. To do this, divide the left-hand page into two columns of equal width. Use the right-hand column for the reworking of class notes and the left-hand column for text notes on the same topic.

On-the-Run Action. The five-stage note-taking model may look time-consuming, but it is not. If you use those minutes in the day that are often lost or wasted for the purpose of reworking and reviewing your notes, the job will be done, leaving large blocks of time to devote to such things as the reading of assigned material. By daily reworking and frequently reviewing your class notes, cumulative learning will take place and the time needed before exams to do a last, thorough review of all the material will be reduced. All this yields the most important benefit—better grades.

MASTERING THE TEXT

The most challenging task most students face is reading, learning, and remembering the material in the textbook. Text material can be long, complex, sometimes confusing, and often highly technical. It can seem as though the more you read, the more there is to learn and the less you understand. Close the book and everything you've just read evaporates from your memory. If you feel like this, just remember—you are not alone. Every student feels this way. However, there are effective ways to maximize your learning and memory and maybe even reduce the time it takes to do this.

Many different study systems have been devised to aid in the mastery of textbook material, and each has worked for some students. The model presented here is a combination of what I think are the best elements of the multitude of systems and the best one for dealing with the subject matter in this text.

TEXT NOTATION

Getting the most from a lecture requires active listening. The same active process applies to the reading of assigned text. There are a number of techniques that promote active reading. A good study system such as the PURR method presented in this chapter is one part of the process. But a good study system can be enhanced by reading with a pencil. Making text notations will help you concentrate and also make future review of the material more productive.

There are three notation systems:
- Highlight/underline
- Marginal notation
- Written text notes

Each of these notation systems has certain advantages and disadvantages. No single one will work perfectly all the time. Just as you must use different techniques to meet the different needs of your patients, you also need to use different techniques of text notation to meet the different needs you have as a learner. First, though, let's discuss some *general* guidelines that apply to the different systems of text notation.

Read First

Before you begin to make any text notations, you must first read the material. The objective of text notations is to identify the important ideas, facts, and terms just as this is the objective of listening during a lecture. If you attempt to mark text while reading it for the first time, everything will seem important and you'll find yourself making far too many notations or highlighting far too much material.

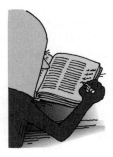

Be Selective

Be very selective. The objective of text notation is much like that of taking notes during a lecture—to pick out the important ideas for immediate learning and for future review. If you have ever looked at a used textbook, you are sure to have seen one in which the previous owner has highlighted nearly every line on some pages. Excessive marking means the reader was not discerning the important ideas as he or she was reading. If you are taking separate handwritten notes, you should limit what you write down to the major headings and subheadings, important and unfamiliar vocabulary, and no more than two sentences of personal notes for each paragraph. The object is not to rewrite the chapter but to distill out the important information. If you are highlighting, limit the material marked to no

Copyright © 2002 by Mosby, Inc. All rights reserved.

more than 20% to 25% of the total material. This is not to say you must impose this limit on every paragraph, but it should be an overall goal.

Text Conventions

As you read and prepare for making text notations, be aware of certain conventions used throughout the text. These are very useful in helping the reader focus on what the authors consider important. By now you have noticed the use of headings in this chapter. Look back at some of them and you will also notice that they are styled differently—some are all capitals; others have only the first letter of each word capitalized. These represent main topics and subtopics. Now look at Chapter 21 in the student text. Examine the way headings and bold facing draw your eyes to certain words, phrases, and portions of the page. These are text conventions provided by the authors to help you understand the organization of the material and the relationship between the material. Other text conventions that you should note are numbered lists, bulleted lists, special display material, and the like.

Language Conventions

Another important aspect of text notation is to become language-sensitive. In a class lecture, when you hear a professor say, for instance, "One of the most important first-generation anesthetics was . . ." the words *most important* are a direct cue that this is an important point for your notes. The same type of cuing often occurs in the text. The authors want to make certain that their important ideas are communicated to you, the reader. Because the authors cannot speak to you face to face, however, they must rely on a certain written style to get important points across. This means that you must become aware of that style so you can identify these important ideas. For example, in Chapter 9, the sentence "Opioids can be classified into four main categories" has the phrase "four main categories," which is the author's way of telling you not only what is coming but also what you should be taking note of.

Later in the same chapter a paragraph begins with the phrase "The most significant effects . . . ." Whenever an author uses words or phrases such as these, it tells you that something important is being discussed. When you highlight text, phrases such as "most important," "four main categories," and "most significant" are the cues you should look for to help identify the most important information. The combination of text conventions and language conventions helps to make the reading and marking of text more successful.

How to Highlight and Underline

Highlighting is a very effective technique for studying and reviewing material. However, you must be very careful when doing it because it is all too easy to highlight text indiscriminately. Text marking is done to help in future review. This means that text marking is a personal process and should be done to point up only the most important information.

It is absolutely essential that you read meaningful blocks of text before you do any marking. A meaningful block may be as little as a single paragraph, but never less. It may be as much as an entire chapter. In a text such as *Pharmacology and the Nursing Process*, in which the material is highly technical and challenging, it is unlikely that you will want to read more than a section of the chapter at a time before going back to highlight.

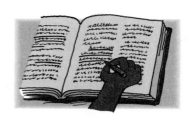

Look at Chapter 11; the first paragraph mentions the italicized terms *sedatives* and *hypnotics*. As you read this paragraph the first time, do not mark anything. Instead read for a general understanding of the content. After this, go back to the beginning of the section and note the following language conventions: "divided," "standard definition," "however," "in addition," "is defined," and "four distinct stages." These are all words and phrases that point up important information that needs to be highlighted. You may not actually need to highlight all the information flagged by these words and phrases. Some is probably already familiar to you because of earlier courses you have taken or earlier chapters you have read in this text. Don't complicate things by highlighting information you have already mastered. At the same time, the repetition of earlier material emphasizes its importance.

Review
When

How soon after you have done some form of text notation should you review what you have highlighted? Ideally it should begin within 24 to 48 hours after the initial learning has occurred. Psychologists

Copyright © 2002 by Mosby, Inc. All rights reserved.

have studied learning, memory, and forgetting and have found that we forget approximately 50% of what we learn after the first day or two. Therefore, the sooner you begin to review, the easier it is to move learning from short-term memory (quickly learned and quickly forgotten) to long-term memory.

How

The process for reviewing any text notations follows the same general principles that apply to lecture notes. The intent is to make your review an active process in which real learning takes place. For example, if you have written questions in the text's margins, try to answer these questions without rereading the text. If you are able to answer the question to your satisfaction, then move on to the next question. If you have highlighted terms and definitions, cover the definition and try to define the term without looking at the text. If you are able to do this, you are effectively moving material into long-term memory. If you can't define the term, then read the text definition. However, don't just look at the words. As you read, think about the meaning and think about strategies you might use to help you remember the term and definition the next time. The key is always to focus on being an active learner.

How Often

How often you review is a personal matter, and there are no rules for determining this precisely. The best way is to be aware of your success, or lack of it, in the current review session. If you do very well at recalling information, then you can probably wait 3 to 4 days for the next review. If the review goes okay, then the next session should take place within 2 days. If you find yourself reviewing your own notations with little understanding and limited memory, then the next review should take place the following day. Each time you review, it will get easier and faster, and as you practice this approach to reviewing your text notations, you will gradually acquire a good sense of how often you need to review to maintain mastery of the material.

PREPARING FOR EXAMS

Test anxiety. Test stress. Test panic. Every student has some experience with this. For some it is a mild anxiety that arises immediately preceding the test; for others it is a stress that begins to build 2 or 3 days before the exam. In the worst instance, it is test panic that hits during the test and causes a near total memory block. Some level of anxiety is perfectly normal. I don't believe it is possible to go into any testing situation absolutely calm and relaxed. Your knowledge and ability are being assessed and graded. Tests *are* important, both in the short term, from the standpoint of grades and successful completion of this course, and also in the long term, from the standpoint of completing the program and getting your degree and eventually the job you want.

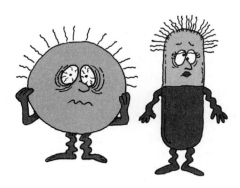

It is easy enough to say that test anxiety is normal, but it does not make it any easier to deal with, and too much anxiety can lead to your making mistakes that can be avoided. You need to start off preparing for exams with the realization that you will feel anxious, but there are things you can do to lower your level of anxiety and improve your performance.

The first and most important rule in preparing for exams is a very simple one: Spend at least 15 minutes every day (Saturdays, Sundays, and holidays included) in reviewing the "old" material. The more time you can find for this each day, the better, but spend at least 15 minutes. This one action will do more to reduce test anxiety than anything else you do. The more time you devote to reviewing past material learned, the more confident you will feel about your knowledge of the topic. This confidence will accompany you into the classroom on the exam day, and it will help you get the kind of test score you want and are capable of. Just remember—start the review process on the first day of the semester and do some review every single day until the final exam.

On-the-Run Action. Study class notes, study vocabulary cards, review highlighted sections of chapters, or meet with your study partner and have a 15-minute quiz session.

Copyright © 2002 by Mosby, Inc. All rights reserved.

Aspects of Preparing for Exams
Materials

Studying for exams requires that you focus on all resource materials. You have the assigned readings in the textbook and class notes to study. In addition, you may have many supplemental materials, such as course handouts, to study. All of this material may be the source of test questions. When doing your ongoing reviews, don't spend all your time on class notes and ignore the assigned readings until a day or two before the exam. One day devote your review time to text materials, and on the next, review class handouts from the previous class. It is also always best to review the notes from the previous class meeting before the next meeting.

Exam Questions

There are several things to consider about the exam proper and the types of questions it will contain. What kind of an exam are you preparing for? Will the test consist entirely of multiple-choice questions? Will it have true-or-false items? Will there be matching, short-answer, or essay questions? You should not study any differently for a multiple-choice exam than you should for a short-answer or essay exam. However, knowing the type or types of questions that will be on the test will help you to develop a strategy for quizzing yourself.

For example, if you know the test will consist of multiple-choice questions, then as you do your review, think of the kinds of questions you would ask if you were composing the test. Consider what would be a good question, what would be the right answer, and what would be other answers that would appear right but would in fact be incorrect. Also consider priority of actions because the best answer may be in the identification of the first or most important nursing action.

If you know the test will contain some short-answer or essay questions, the same rule applies. Make up your own test questions and then rehearse the answers to them. Also consider where the ideas for questions come from. They will most likely come from the chapter headings and glossaries in your textbook and from the topic labels you noted in the left-hand column of your class notes during the reworking phase.

When and Where

We have already stressed the need to review every day, but you must also consider the time of day, the location, and how long the review session is going to be. These also have an important bearing on how efficient and effective the review process is. Reviewing can be done in relatively short periods of time, unlike the large blocks of time needed to read chapters. Look carefully at your daily schedule and note those small amounts of time between classes, after lunch, while waiting for the washer to finish the spin cycle, or during whatever activities might yield small blocks of time. Learn to use these times for review. If you have five blocks of 10 minutes each in a day and you use three of them for review, you have just gained 30 minutes and done a lot of review.

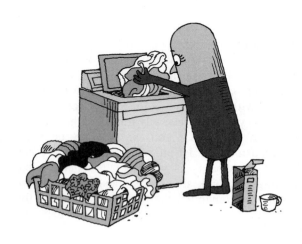

Where you do this review is important, too. Some students claim they can study in the middle of a rock concert, though I have some doubts about this, whereas others need a quiet environment. Whatever the setting, don't pick a place for test preparation that has built-in distractions. If you cannot resist the lure of the television, then you should study in a room without a TV. If family members are a distraction, then try to find more time at school or at work to use for study. Study in the school library or an empty classroom, but stay away from the student center or cafeteria where the distractions are plentiful.

How to Prepare

Although the time and place are important aspects of preparing for exams, the most important aspect is the way in which you study. The best learning takes place when you are actively engaged with the material. Rereading text material, handouts, and notes is not the best way to study because rereading may not foster the active mental processing and assimilation of material. Because the best way to prepare for an exam is to take one, try to make your review a pretend exam.

Copyright © 2002 by Mosby, Inc. All rights reserved.

Reviewing Class Notes

Look at your class notes. If you have been using the split-page model described earlier, you have made your own topic headings in the left-hand column beside the class notes. Cover the class notes and turn each heading into one or more questions. Think carefully about the answers and then answer the questions *aloud.* By answering questions aloud, you are forcing yourself to think about what you know and organizing that knowledge in the way that is most meaningful to you. If you can answer your own questions, then you have demonstrated that you know the material, and there is no immediate need to reread that section of notes. If you cannot answer one of your own questions, then you know you need to review this material more intensively. Uncover the notes, and read the pertinent ones. You are now using your review time very effectively because instead of just rereading everything, which invites boredom, or worse yet, daydreaming, the rereading is directed at the material you are unsure of. The result of all this is more efficient use of your time and more effective learning.

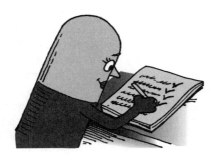

Reviewing the Textbook

The technique you used for studying your class notes will also work for studying text material. As already mentioned, in this book the authors have provided you with a variety of features that can help enormously in this process. First, look at the objectives at the beginning of each chapter to be studied. Even if you have been assigned only small portions of the chapter, it is still important to consider the objectives for the chapter as a whole. Ask yourself whether you have met these objectives. This is a quick way of assessing how much review may be necessary. If you feel confident that you have accomplished most of the objectives, then the review should go quickly. If you feel uncertain about many of them, then you know the review is going to take more time.

The next task is to consider the topic headings and language conventions. Use them in the same way as you have used the labels in your notes. Turn them into questions and answer them aloud. If you can answer them, then there is no need to reread. If you can't, then you will need to reread the pertinent text.

Again, this way of reviewing is focusing your time and energy mostly where it is needed—on the material you have not yet mastered. Each time you review text (or class notes), the sections of material you reread may differ. This is to be expected. You cannot remember everything forever. But, if you spend time each day doing this type of review, you will remember more and more and for longer and longer periods.

Reviewing Terminology

One aspect of nursing that can seem overwhelming is the terminology. It is highly technical and very specialized. Learning it poses the same kind of challenge as learning a foreign language. In fact, it very nearly is a foreign language. However, in order to master the concepts and ideas, it is imperative that the terms be mastered. One of the best ways to go about doing this is to use a technique you probably learned in grade school—flash cards. Put the term on one side of a 3×5 notecard and the definition or other essential information about the term on the back. Group cards together with terms that have common word elements, such as *cardio,* or that have common concepts, such as all terms having to do with renal function or blood pressure. The more relationships you can establish between words, the easier it will be to learn and remember them.

On-the-Run Action. Get in the habit of carrying a deck of 10 to 15 of these cards with you all the time. When you have a few minutes, review as many cards as time allows. Sometimes start with the term side of the card and try to recall what is written on the back. Other times look at the definitions on the back of the card, and try to recall the term. Don't focus exclusively on term-to-definition learning because you may be given definitions or some variation of them on the exam and asked to provide the terms.

TAKING EXAMS

This is it. The culmination of all your work—lectures, notes, flash cards, textbook readings, and handouts. First and foremost, relax. I know that is easier said than done, but it is important to try to relax because test anxiety interferes with test performance. If you have put to use the learning

Copyright © 2002 by Mosby, Inc. All rights reserved.

techniques described in this chapter, you should be ready for the exam. You have mastered the material and you can do well on the exam.

Besides these learning techniques, however, there are also techniques for dealing with the various types of exam questions, and these are discussed in this section. None of these strategies can guarantee a 10-point jump on the test score. Only the degree to which you have mastered the material can make that sort of difference. But, each of the strategies described in this section may only help you answer one or two questions correctly that you might otherwise have missed. If a particular test strategy adds 2 points to your score, it is a valuable strategy, because small differences in test scores can have a greater effect on your final grade. These test-taking strategies are not intended to replace regular study and mastery, however. They are intended to enhance your test performance. If you use these strategies, you will see a positive gain in your test performance.

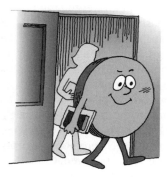

However, before discussing these specific strategies, I want to focus first on more general strategies for taking tests.

General Test Strategies

Be Prepared. As has been emphasized throughout this chapter, studying for an exam begins the first day of class and continues every day of the semester. If you have been doing regular study and review, then you are prepared.

The Night Before. Do a thorough review of the material to be covered on the exam. Do not put in an all-night cram session. Spend 2 or 3 hours reviewing. Focus on facts, terms, and concepts that have been stressed in both the classroom and in the textbook. These are the items that are most likely going to be on the test. Use the oral question-and-answer technique described throughout this chapter. Don't concentrate exclusively on the things you have had trouble mastering, however. Also spend

some time quickly and briefly reviewing the things you do know. Focusing totally on what you don't know will increase test anxiety. This will also tend to obscure the material that has been mastered. Most of your review time needs to be spent on trouble areas, but balance it out with some review of areas you are confident about.

Don't try to study for 3 hours straight. If your schedule permits it, spread out this last review session over several small sessions. Put in an hour in the afternoon, then take a break and do something that is a reward (remember the gold stars and M&Ms). Then come back and spend another hour in review. Take another break, and hit the books one more time. Then, YOU ARE DONE! Watch a little television or enjoy some other pastime, then get a good night's sleep. Fatigue interferes with test performance almost as much as anxiety.

Exam Day. The test is at 10 A.M. and you get to school at 8. You have a class at 8 but an hour free between 9 and 10. *Don't study for the exam during that time.* The temptation will be great, but resist it. Studying right before an exam only creates additional stress because the tendency is to focus on those areas you are worried about. The more you worry about them, the more likely you are to drive the material you know well out of your memory. If you have free time before the exam, do something completely unrelated to the course. Take a walk. Go to the library and read a magazine (and not a nursing journal). Stop by the cafeteria and have a cup of coffee or a soda. A few minutes before the test time, head for the classroom. Make sure you have two pens or pencils, an eraser, blank paper, your text, and your class notes. There is nothing worse than discovering, just as the test is starting, that you don't have some essential tool for the test. Don't get to the room 15 or 20 minutes early. If you do, you are likely to sit there and fret and stew about the exam, and that also produces test anxiety. If you know the material, you don't need to be anxious.

Exam Time. This is it. The teacher passes out the exam. All your work and preparation are about to pay off. But, don't just leap into the test. Take a couple of minutes to put yourself in a frame of mind for doing well on the test. At this point, you have a perfect test score—you haven't answered any questions incorrectly yet. It is likely you will get some answers wrong, but don't start out by making mistakes that cost you points you shouldn't have lost.

First, look over the entire test. Don't read it, but turn the pages and look at a question here and a question there. How many items are there on the test? Are all the questions of one type, or is there a mixture of types? Knowing in advance the length of the test and the types of questions helps you plan your strategy for taking the test.

Copyright © 2002 by Mosby, Inc. All rights reserved.

Second, read the directions. This is the first opportunity you have to make a mistake that could cost points. I include some true-or-false items on all my tests. On the first test in the course, my written directions tell students to use block capitals "F" and "T" to mark their answers. For most students this is the way true-or-false marking has always been done, and it is what they expect. By the time of the next test, we have covered test-taking strategies in the class, and I have stressed the importance of reading the directions. On this next test the written directions tell students to use a plus symbol to indicate true and a minus symbol to indicate false. I say nothing about the directions; I leave it to the students to read and follow them. After 20 years of teaching, I have not yet had a class in which every student has followed the true-or-false directions on the second test. I only take 2 points off for failure to follow these directions, but consider that the difference between an A and a B can be only 2 points. Read the directions. It doesn't take much time, and it could save you 2 points, or more!

Now you are ready to start answering the questions. If the test consists of all one type of question, then start with the first question. But if the test has multiple-choice, true-or-false, and short-essay questions, you have to decide where it is best for you to start. If you find essay questions easy to do, then maybe you should start with these. There is no reason you have to begin with the multiple-choice ones. On the other hand, if you find essay questions a challenge, then don't start with them. Begin the test in a way that will give you confidence.

Wherever you choose to begin, there is one more thing to consider before you start. You have looked through the test and know the number and type of questions. You now need to plan how to complete the test in the time allowed. For example, if the test has 50 multiple-choice questions and the time limit is 40 minutes, then you know you will have to average a little better than one item per minute. Obviously you will need to allocate more time to essay questions if they are on the exam. In addition, as you are taking the test, glance at your watch or the classroom clock occasionally to make sure you are not losing time or going too quickly. If you have been working for 15 minutes and have done 20 items, there is no problem. If you have completed 25 items, you are well ahead of schedule and can slow down if you feel the need to. If, on the other hand, you have only completed 10 or 11 items by that time, you are moving a little slowly and may end up being under real pressure to finish all the items before the time runs out.

If you are answering questions quickly and are confident that the answers are right, don't worry about being ahead of schedule. But, spending too much time on individual questions can find you trying to decide the answers to the last questions quickly, and this increases your chances of making errors. Planning a strategy for finishing the test within the time allowed helps you maintain a sharp focus on the task and enables you to do the best job possible.

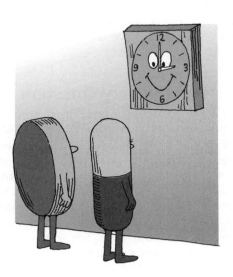

Answering the Questions

Now that the planning aspect is completed, you can begin answering the questions. Start with the first question or with those types of questions you feel most confident answering. Wherever you choose to start, there is a strategy you can use that can improve your test performance. Read the question *carefully,* and if you know the answer, indicate it and move to the next question. If you cannot immediately think of the answer, give it a few seconds of thought. If the answer comes, indicate it and move on. If the answer still doesn't come or if the question is confusing, then skip to the next question. In the first pass through the exam, answer what you know and skip what you don't. There are two important benefits to doing this.

First, answering the questions you are sure of increases your confidence and saves time. You are sure of your answers, and you don't have to be concerned with these questions anymore. And because they take little time to complete, this is buying you time to devote to the questions you have more difficulty with.

Second, because the subjects of the questions on a particular exam are related, the answers to questions you have skipped may be provided by other questions on the test. Or a later question may trigger recall of the correct answer.

Copyright © 2002 by Mosby, Inc. All rights reserved.

Either way, skipping questions you are unsure of offers one more opportunity to get the correct answer.

After you have gone through the entire test answering the questions you are confident of, go back to the items you skipped. But first check the time so you know how much time you have left to answer these questions. On this second pass through the exam you will often be surprised at how many questions you now can answer that were a complete blank before.

Answer Every Question

Never, never, never leave questions unanswered. A question without an answer is the same as a wrong answer, and worse than that, you haven't even given yourself a chance to get it right, and get the added points on your score. Again and again I tell students this rule, and they continue to turn in tests with unanswered questions. When I ask them why they've left questions blank, they inevitably say it was because they weren't sure of the answer or didn't know it and thought it was better not to guess. GO AHEAD AND GUESS. You've studied for the test and you should know the material well. You're not making a random guess based on no information. You are guessing based on what you have learned and your best assessment of the question. Once again, remember that the points you lose by not answering versus the 2 points you stand to get by making an educated guess can really make a difference in your score.

Turn In the Exam

When you've answered *all* the questions on the test, turn it in. A quick check to make sure you haven't skipped any items is okay, but don't start back through the test second-guessing yourself. Second-guessing at this point is likely to spark the desire to start changing answers, and there is nothing worse than changing right answers to wrong. Have confidence in your own knowledge and let go of the test. If you are the first person to complete a test but are sure of what you did, then turn it in. At the same time, don't let what others in the class are doing affect your test strategy. If you are the last person to turn the test in, it doesn't mean you know less than those who were faster. It simply means that you are a careful, thoughtful test taker.

Strategies for Specific Types of Questions

For each type of question there are particular strategies you can use that can help prevent incor-

rect responses. Many times students miss questions not because of a lack of information but because of a poor strategy. Sometimes the error stems from misreading a question, for instance, overlooking a key word such as "not," or from choosing an answer that doesn't quite fit the question asked. Errors like these can be costly. Expect to find some questions on a test that you don't remember the answer to or that are worded in a confusing way. A perfect test score is a great goal, but be realistic and accept the fact that perfect scores may be few and far between. At the same time, don't lose points because of careless, and preventable, errors.

Strategy for Multiple-Choice Questions

Multiple-choice questions (sometimes called *multiple-guess questions*) can be very challenging. All too often students think that they will recognize the right answer when they see it or that the right answer will somehow stand out from the other choices. This is a dangerous misconception. The more carefully the question is constructed, the more each of the choices should seem like the correct response. There are a number of things that the successful student can do to improve performance on multiple-choice questions.

Multiple-Choice Terminology. Before discussing the strategies for analyzing multiple-choice questions, it is important to understand each part of a question and its purpose.

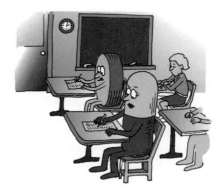

First, there is the question stem. This is the complete question that one, or more, of the response choices will answer.

EXAMPLE:

Why did the United States annex Hawaii from Spain?

Notice that this could just as easily be a short-answer question. In this case the stem is a complete sentence that should be answered by one of the

Copyright © 2002 by Mosby, Inc. All rights reserved.

response choices. The stem can also be an incomplete statement that one, or more, of the response choices completes correctly.

EXAMPLE:

The likelihood of a drug's therapeutic effects increases dramatically when:

This statement is incomplete, and you must pick out the response choice that best completes it.

A second part of multiple-choice questions is distractors. These are the response choices that do not best answer or complete the stem. They are known as *distractors* because that is their purpose, to distract you from the best choice. Good distractors are usually very similar to the best choice. If you have not studied enough, a good distractor will be a very tempting choice, but you must reduce the allure of distractors.

The third and final part of all multiple-choice questions is the best choice. This is the choice you want to pick. Notice I have said "best choice." In many multiple-choice questions there may be more than one response choice that appears to answer the stem, and the differences between the responses may be slight. Your task is therefore to identify the choice that *best* responds to the stem, not necessarily the only right answer.

Strategies for Analysis. The most reliable way to ensure that you select the correct response to a multiple-choice question is to recall it. Depend on your learning and memory to furnish the answer to the question. To do this, read the stem, and then STOP! Don't look at the response options yet. Try to recall what you know and, based on this, what you would give as the answer. After you have taken a few seconds to do this, then look at *all* the choices and select the one that most nearly matches the answer you recalled. It is important that you consider *all* the choices and not just choose the first option that seems to fit the answer you recall. Remember the distractors. Choice B may look okay but choice D may be worded in such a way that makes D a slightly better choice. If you don't weigh all the choices, you are not maximizing your chances of correctly answering each question.

Once you've decided on an answer, there is one more important step before you mark it. Look at the stem again. Does your choice answer the question that was asked? If the question stem asks "why," be sure the response you have chosen is a reason. If the question stem is singular, then be sure the option is singular, and the same for plural stems and plural responses. Many times, checking to make sure the choice makes sense in relation to the stem will reveal the correct answer.

This is the most reliable technique to use for answering multiple-choice questions. If you do this for every multiple-choice question on the test, your accuracy rate will be very high, and you will not need any further strategy. Unfortunately, however, recall doesn't always work, and when it doesn't, there are some additional strategies you can apply to improve your chances of picking the correct answer.

Recognition and Elimination. It will happen. You read the stem and you can't recall the answer. Don't panic; all is not lost. It just takes a little more work and thought, but you can still answer the item correctly. Read each of the choice options carefully. Usually at least one of them will be clearly wrong. Eliminate this one from consideration. Now you have reduced the number of response choices from four to three and improved the odds. Continue to analyze the options. If you can eliminate one more choice in a four-option question, you have reduced the odds to 50/50, the same as the odds of random guessing in true-or-false questions, and there are still some strategies that will help you pick the best choice. In addition, while you are eliminating the wrong choices, recall often occurs. One of the options may serve as a trigger that causes you to remember what a few seconds ago had seemed completely forgotten.

LOOK-ALIKE ANSWERS. After you have eliminated one or more choices, you may discover that two of the options are very similar. This can be very helpful because it may mean that one of these look-alike answers is the best choice and the other is a very good distractor. Test both of these options against the stem. Ask yourself which one completes the incomplete statement grammatically and which one answers the question more fully and completely? The option that best completes or answers the stem is the one you should choose. Here, too, pause for a few seconds, give your brain time to reflect, and recall may occur.

ABSOLUTES. Absolute words and phrases can also help you determine the correct answer to a multiple-choice item. If a choice option contains an absolute (for example, *none, never, must, cannot*), be very cautious. Remember there aren't many things in this world that are absolute, and in an area as complex as pharmacology, an absolute as an option may be reason to eliminate it from consideration as the best choice. This is only a guideline, however, and should not be taken to be true 100% of the time, but it can help you reduce the number of choices.

NEGATIVES AND EXCEPTIONS. In the stem "A drug reaction to _____ could include all but which of these symptoms?" the phrase "all but" tells you to choose the response that is an exception. ALL BUT ONE of the choice options is a symptom. In this case the option that is not a symptom is the best choice. If you look at the options and see

Copyright © 2002 by Mosby, Inc. All rights reserved.

several that seem correct, look at the stem again. It may be that you have overlooked an exception phrase such as "all but" or "all but one."

A similar stem wording that can throw you off is a negative or negative prefix. The stem "It is generally NOT a good idea to administer adult dosages to . . ." is asking you to select the answer that names the inappropriate, not appropriate, recipient of a medication. The word *not* helps identify the answer.

All these strategies can help you analyze the response choices so that you have the best possible chance of selecting the correct choice. When you are ready to mark the answer, keep in mind that the final step is always to test your response against the stem.

If, after you've tried all these strategies, you find yourself still unable to choose a response, there is one final strategy. Ask the instructor for clarification of the question. There is nothing to lose by asking and everything to gain. The worst that can happen is that the instructor will tell you that he or she cannot answer your question. The best that can happen is that the instructor will rephrase the question in a way that resolves the problem for you.

When asking for such clarification, try to phrase your question in a way that encourages a response. Don't simply state that you don't understand this question. This is generally not the approach that invites an answer. If you are having trouble with a term in the stem or response choices, ask for a definition. If there is a phrase that is unclear or a response choice that is confusing, ask for clarification. Anything you do to make your question more specific increases the likelihood the instructor will answer it.

After all other avenues have been exhausted, remember the final rule. NEVER LEAVE A QUESTION UNANSWERED. Even if answering is no more than an educated guess on your part, go ahead and mark an answer. You might be right, but if you leave it blank, you will certainly be wrong and lose precious points.

Strategy for Short-Answer and Essay Questions

Short-answer and essay questions tend to be either loved or hated. Some students prefer this kind of question and are very confident in their ability to perform well on them. Others react to them with anything from mild dislike to intense anxiety. There seem to be very few students who have a neutral attitude toward them. Whichever way you feel, the strategies in this section will help you improve your performance on such questions.

Before getting into the strategy proper, I want to explain that I am discussing the strategy for answering short-answer and essay questions together because both types of questions require careful thought and planning before you write an answer. I am also doing this because I think it is helpful to get into the habit of regarding short-answer questions as short-essay questions. Too often students lose points on short-answer questions by being too brief. A short answer should usually consist of three or four sentences, but frequently students interpret "short answer" to mean four or five words.

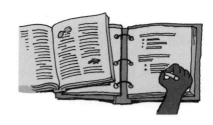

To start off answering these questions, you must analyze the question carefully and then frame a response that will fully answer it. Assume the reader, in this case the course instructor, doesn't know anything and you have to explain it all. Short-answer and essay questions require you to show what you know. Don't assume the instructor can read your mind or read between the lines of your response to discern what you knew but didn't include. It is better to have a little more than was needed in your answer than not enough. Extra information won't hurt, but missing information will always cost points. Once again, remember that the idea is to gain a point here and there throughout the test, with the end result being a higher score and a better grade for the course.

Two Key Issues. *First,* in writing answers to these questions, it is essential to answer exactly the question that is asked. This means that you must understand the question before you do any writing. Unlike true-or-false and multiple-choice questions, which you should try to answer using every strategy before seeking help, when it comes to these questions, you should ask for help before doing anything. The first opportunity you have to lose points in an essay question occurs with the first reading of the question. If you misread the question, you may write an excellent answer but not the right one. Such a mistake can be costly.

Second, a good answer must be organized so that it is clear and logical to the reader. Do not read a question and start writing down whatever ideas

Copyright © 2002 by Mosby, Inc. All rights reserved.

spring to mind. Spend a minute or two thinking and planning the structure of the answer so that your ideas are clearly stated and the supporting details relate directly to each idea. Your instructor, the reader, will have a very difficult time grading your essay if he or she has to read it two or three times to figure out what you were trying to say. Organization and clarity of expression really pay off in essay exams.

Five Steps to Good Essay Answers

Read Questions Carefully. As was discussed earlier, misreading the question can result in a high-quality answer that does not address the question asked. Read and think about the question's major focus. Do not jump on the first familiar phrase or term and start writing without further thought.

Decision Step. Telling you to read the question carefully is good advice, but without some strategy to apply to the reading it might be very difficult advice to carry out. Here is a strategy to help you read carefully and begin to plan your answer. Look at the question as you read, and identify the words and phrases that tell you what to do. There are some standard "what to do" words and phrases that are used consistently in essay questions, such as *discuss, compare, contrast, explain, tell why,* and *analyze.* Circle each of these words or phrases as you read the question. The second part of the decision step is to underline *what* you are to write about. This circling and underlining will force a careful reading of the question and help you begin the process of organizing the answer. The sample question that follows is marked to show the circle and underline strategy.

SAMPLE QUESTION:

(Discuss) the ways in which pediatric and geri-atric patients are alike in determining appropriate dosage. (Explain) why adult dosage may be inap-propriate *and* the dangers in using adult dosage on these special populations.

Quick Written Outline. Before you start writing your answer, take a few minutes to organize the points you want to cover. This should not be an elaborate outline with roman numerals, capital letters, and Arabic numbers, but rather a quick

sketch of the question and the points you want to make in the answer. The circle and underline step will help to make this easy to do.

EXAMPLE OUTLINE*:
Discuss
- Pediatric/geriatric patients similarity to drug dose
  - Body weight factor
  - Organ function

Explain
- Reasons adult dose inappropriate
  - Drugs not tested on pediatric and geriatric population
- Dangers of adult dose
  - Possible organ damage
  - Increased absorption and possible side effects

An outline like this will organize your ideas, speed your writing, and ensure that you are answering the question asked.

*This is a model of the process of the Decision and Outline Steps. It is not to be viewed as an accurate outline of pharmacologic content.

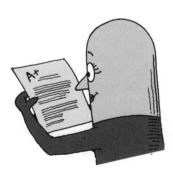

Write an Answer. With the question analyzed and a quick outline in place, it is time to put your answer on paper.

Basic Structure of Essay Responses. One way to think about the short answer/essay is to consider it as an in-class composition assignment with an assigned topic. Every rule that composition teachers insist on in writing assignments should be used in writing essay answers.

Any answer of more than four or five sentences should follow the basic three-part essay structure of introduction, body, and conclusion.

Introduction. There should be an introduction. It should not be more than one or two sentences in

Copyright © 2002 by Mosby, Inc. All rights reserved.

length, but it serves to tell the reader what you are going to present in your answer. There is a relatively simple way to write an essay introduction. State the question positively and add a few words that show the main points you intend to make in your answer.

EXAMPLE INTRODUCTION:

Pediatric and geriatric patients have a number of similarities that must be considered in determining drug dosage. Two of the most important are body weight and organ function, and these factors can make adult dosages inappropriate for these two populations.

These two sentences tell the reader exactly what you plan to discuss. From this point on, it becomes your task to explain why those two are important and how they affect drug dosage. You have told the reader what to expect, and you have begun to organize your answer.

Body. This is the most important part of any essay answer. In it you want to state the ideas, concepts, and points that you believe answer the question. These should be stated clearly and positively. Don't ramble on trying to cover all the possible variations that might fit into an answer. Decide on the most important, most significant points you have to make. Then state them and support and explain with relevant details that show how and why your points answer the question. In short answer questions where three to five sentences are expected, drop the introduction and conclusion, and put all your energy into a clear, concise body.

Conclusion. There should be a concluding sentence or two to let the reader know that you have finished. Like the introduction, it should be brief and, like the introduction, it is relatively easy to write. Restate the question and summarize the key points made in your answer.

EXAMPLE CONCLUSION:

It is clear that geriatric and pediatric patients are very similar in their response to drug dosages. Clearly the factors of body weight and organ function will play a major role in determining the appropriate dosages for these two groups.

Read the Answer. The writing is completed. Before you turn in the paper, take another minute or two and read over what you have written. Look for errors that would make the reader pause, question what you have said, or be unable to read a word or phrase. Sometimes the mind works much faster than the pen, and a word or phrase is left out in writing. Use the caret (^) and insert the word or phrase

where it belongs. If your writing got a little sloppy and a word is hard to read, cross it out and print it clearly right above. Proofreading and correcting small errors like these will make the answer easier to read and understand. Anything that contributes to the overall quality of an answer will influence the grade in a positive manner. You won't have time to rewrite an answer, but you should correct obvious errors.

Strategy for True-or-False Questions

True-or-false items outwardly appear to be fairly simple. After all, the statement is either true or false. The odds are 50/50, and if all else fails, a coin toss can decide the issue. Appearances are deceiving, however, and true-or-false questions can be very challenging to answer. Good test strategy applies to all types of questions because the object is to get the best score you can, and remember, this represents the *total* points for all the correct answers.

Read the Question. Reading the question may seem like such an obvious part of all test strategy that it may appear absurd to even be told this. But, if you don't pay careful attention to the wording of true-or-false statements, then you are increasing the odds of making an otherwise avoidable error. Take the time to read and understand the statement. Read it all the way through to the end. Don't jump to conclusions based on half the statement.

Assume the Statement Is True. As you read each true-or-false statement, begin with the assumption that the statement is true. The idea behind this strategy is that it will cause you to read the statement carefully, which will result in your choosing the correct answer. This approach to reading the statement makes the reading an active process because you are then reading to confirm the truth in the statement. You will be analyzing the statement as you read, looking for any information that would contradict or change the statement from true to false. You will also be choosing your answer as you read rather than waiting to the end to decide whether it was true or false. Obviously not every statement will be true, but this step makes you a much more thoughtful reader, and that encourages better test performance.

Remember one other important rule when analyzing true-or-false statements. IF ANY PART OF THE STATEMENT IS FALSE, THEN THE ENTIRE STATEMENT IS FALSE. There may be only one altered word or prefix (such as *un-* or *anti-*) that changes a statement from true to false, but that is all that is required.

Copyright © 2002 by Mosby, Inc. All rights reserved.

Strategies for Analysis. Sometimes, no matter how carefully you have read the question, the answer is not immediately obvious. When that happens, there are a number of strategies you can use to analyze the question. Using these strategies will not guarantee you'll get the correct answer, but they will often help you see something about the statement you might have overlooked and help you to identify the correct answer.

ABSOLUTES AND QUALIFIERS. Absolutes are words such as *none*, *never*, *all*, or *always*. These words mean that there are absolutely no exceptions to the statement. For instance, the statement "All birds fly" means just that. Every bird, past, present, and future, has flown or does fly. If there is or has been just one bird that has not flown or does not fly, then the statement is false. "All" in this statement is an absolute. True-or-false statements that contain such absolutes are usually false. In an area as complex as pharmacology it is unlikely that there are many absolutes. If you are struggling with a question that has you stumped, look for absolute words. They may help you to determine the answer.

On the other hand, there are words that suggest the possibility of exceptions. Such words or phrases are called *qualifiers;* examples of these are *some*, *possibly*, *in most cases*, and *will generally*. "Most birds can fly" is an example of a qualified statement. The word *most* tells you that some not precisely specified number of the total of all birds can fly. This makes it more probable that the statement is true.

STATED IN THE NEGATIVE. A true-or-false statement that is rendered in the negative can be very difficult to answer. To use the earlier example, "It is not true that all birds can fly" is such a statement. The word *not* in this statement can make it much more complex to read and answer. There is a relatively simple way to deal with this type of statement. Read it as though the negative was not included, so that it becomes "It is true that all birds can fly." This statement is clearly false. Because the word *not* reverses the meaning of the statement, this makes the statement "It is not true that all birds can fly" true. Simply put, if the statement is true without the negative, then it becomes false with the negative. Vice versa, if it is false without the negative, then it is true with the negative.

STRINGS. A string is a true-or-false statement that requires careful attention. It is a statement that contains a list of several words or phrases, but often one or more of the words or phrases is false. It is easy to read the statement and see that the first two or three words or phrases are true but then to overlook the one that is incorrect, with the consequence that you mark the answer as true when it is actually false. An example of a string is: "Many warm weather crops, such as tomatoes, can be grown year-round in southern California, southern Florida, South America, and South Dakota." As you read this statement, it is easy to be lured by the words *southern* and *South* into thinking the statement is true without noting the fact that South Dakota is a northern state with fairly harsh winters, and there are parts of South America where the climate is very cold. The statement is false, but the string can trick you into thinking the statement is true.

These strategies for analyzing true-or-false items can help you increase the number of correct answers. They are not intended, however, to replace study and learning because the best way to perform well on any test is to know the answers based on your own learning. However, when the answer does not immediately come to mind, apply these strategies. Although they won't necessarily lead to a 10-point difference in your score, they may help you add 2 points to your score. And better scores mean better course grades, and of course, this makes for improved self-confidence and improved chances of success.

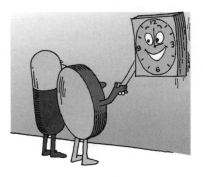

STRATEGIES FOR VOCABULARY DEVELOPMENT

Every specialty and discipline has its own language that must be learned for full mastery to occur. In political science, terms such as *radical, conservative,* and *liberal* and their definitions must be learned and integrated into a person's knowledge of the discipline. The same holds true for psychology and terms such as *behavior modification, operant conditioning,* and *classical conditioning.* Courses such as this one on pharmacology contain extremely complex materials, and terminology is a major component of that complexity. In technologic, scientific, and medical areas, mastering the vocabulary can make the difference between being successful and struggling constantly to understand

Copyright © 2002 by Mosby, Inc. All rights reserved.

the ideas and concepts being presented. Without a thorough mastery of the terminology, it can seem as if you are listening to or reading a foreign language, and your understanding will be severely hampered as a result. It is therefore helpful to adopt some strategies that can make the process of vocabulary development easier and more effective.

Tools

Before describing some specific strategies and techniques to help you master the vocabulary of pharmacology, it is important to consider some of the tools that will help.

Dictionaries

First, it is essential that you have a good current desk reference dictionary. *Current* means the most recent edition of whatever dictionary you choose. A dictionary published 10 or 15 years ago may contain most of what you need, but unless there have been periodic revisions, as shown on the copyright page, it is almost certain to lack some information, and this may cause you problems. When I say *desk reference,* I mean a quality hardbound dictionary and not a condensed or paperback version. Paperbacks are convenient to carry around, but to get the dictionary to this convenient size, some words have been omitted and some definitions have been shortened. This is not what you want. You need the most complete and current edition you can find and afford.

You may or may not need a medical dictionary. You will probably have access to one or more at your college or departmental library. The best way to decide whether you need to invest in such a specialized dictionary is to ask your instructor for his or her advice.

Text Glossary

As soon as you look at any of the remaining chapters in this text, you will discover the glossary. A glossary is nothing more than a text-specific dictionary. It contains the terms and definitions the authors consider essential for a full understanding of the material. The glossary will not necessarily contain every term that is unfamiliar to you. (This is why you need a good dictionary.) Always begin the process of mastering vocabulary by paying particular attention to the glossary and key terms.

Note Cards

Obtain a supply of notecards. Pick the size that best accommodates your handwriting style and size.

But if 5 × 7 cards don't fit into your notebook, pocketbook, or book bag, and this discourages you from carrying them around with you, then use the 3 × 5 cards. Remember, the flash cards these become are one of the best things you can study on the run.

Techniques
Use What You Know

The first strategy to apply in acquiring the vocabulary needed for an understanding of pharmacology is to apply what you already know. When you encounter an unfamiliar word, don't automatically assume you have no idea what it means. Use the knowledge you have already acquired in other nursing courses and throughout your life.

For instance, *psychotherapeutic* appears in the chapter title for Chapter 14. Your first reaction may be that you don't know what it means. But by using what you know, you may be able to make an educated guess as to the meaning of the word without consulting either the text glossary or a dictionary.

This is how you make that educated guess. Consider that the first part of the word is *psycho-*. By this point in your career as a student, you know that *psycho-* refers to the mind. This is a good start. Now consider the next part of the word. The meaning of *therapeutic* may or may not be evident to you, but it should remind you of a simpler word, *therapy,* which constitutes the treatment used to cure or alleviate an illness or a condition. Put "mind" and 'treatment' together, and it would seem that *psychotherapeutic* must refer to the treatment of mental problems.

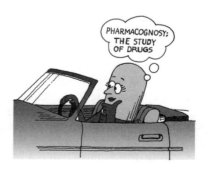

Note, this is an educated guess. It may not be a perfect definition, but it will give you a basis for acquiring a fuller understanding when the term is defined in the glossary or introduced and defined in the text of the chapter. The first sentence in Chapter 14 confirms that this educated guess is very close to the actual meaning: "The term *psychotherapeutics* refers to the therapy of emotional and mental disor-

Copyright © 2002 by Mosby, Inc. All rights reserved.

ders." Using this approach to analyzing the meaning of a word not only confirms that you have a basic understanding of the word but also cultivates a mental link between what you know and the more specific definition provided in the text. Words and their meanings learned in this way are usually easier to grasp and easier to retain. Unfortunately, this technique will not work with some of the terms used in pharmacology because they are so specialized and specific to the field. This calls for the use of other techniques.

Learn the Standard Abbreviations

Make sure as you read that you pay attention to the "shorthand" used. For example, in Chapter 11, the abbreviation *CNS* is used repeatedly. The first time it is presented, the author identifies it as standing for *central nervous system* by putting the abbreviation in parentheses after the term. Thereafter it is used in lieu of the long term. The same thing is done for *REM* in this chapter. It is essential that you learn these abbreviations and recall each, not as a set of meaningless letters, but as a key term that must be mastered.

Establish Relationships

REM is an abbreviation for *rapid eye movements,* and this term refers to a particular stage of sleep. Chapter 11 deals with central nervous system depressants. Relating REM to the focus of this chapter will help you to remember that CNS depressants are used to affect sleep. The idea is to establish a clear relationship between the terms used and the ideas presented in these chapters. Words should not be learned in isolation from the content; otherwise, you may know lots of words and their meanings but not be able to relate them to ideas and content. On tests, you are not likely to be asked to just repeat memorized definitions. Instead you will be asked to integrate these meanings into your answers to questions about nursing practices and applications.

Another important way of relating words to meanings is to link the meanings of closely related terms. The words *hypnotic* and *sedative* are good examples of this. In looking at the meanings in the glossary, you will find that each refers to a certain class of drugs. Both classes of agents affect the CNS, but the agents in each have a somewhat different effect. It is useful to start with the understanding that both affect the CNS but then to appreciate how the terms relate to each other. Sedatives inhibit the CNS but do not cause sleep; hypnotics at

low doses have the same effect, but at higher doses they may induce sleep. In this learning method, you learn meanings by looking at the general similarities and then at the specific differences between terms. In doing this, you have learned both words and should never have any problems relating words to their meanings.

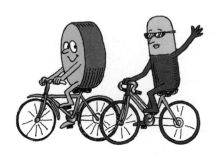

AN INSPIRING CASE STUDY

I wish I could sit down and talk to you about my own somewhat checkered past as a college student. During my first 2 years, I was a very unsuccessful student—unsuccessful to such an extent that the state university I was attending told me at the end of my second year that I would not be allowed to return. My average grade was a dismal D–. There were many factors that contributed to my lack of success, but in retrospect I realize that the biggest single factor responsible was my lack of study skills and learning strategies.

After a 2-year hiatus, I started attending another university as a part-time student. Knowing that I wanted to become a teacher made it imperative that I succeed in college. Over the course of about a year, I invented some strategies to help me succeed. Later I discovered that the strategies I thought I had invented were to be found in many books on study skills. If I had known that, it might have prevented my disastrous first 2 years and certainly would have eliminated the need for me to reinvent them.

The techniques presented in this chapter are not new, original, or magical. They are tried-and-true techniques that thousands of students have used with success. They work. How do I know that? First, they have worked (and continue to work) for me as a student. Second, I have been teaching these ideas for 25 years, first in high school and now for more than 20 years in a community college. Students prove they work by reporting back to me on their success, their improved grades, and even the pleasure they have in being a student.

For myself these tools helped me complete a bachelor's degree, a master's degree, and then a second master's degree. I enjoy being a student because I know I am going to succeed, and I know I

Copyright © 2002 by Mosby, Inc. All rights reserved.

am going to succeed because I know how to learn. It is all here in this chapter. If you use these tools from day one, and use them every day of your student career, you will be successful. Remember the line from *Star Wars*: "May the force be with you." These tools are the "force" that will ensure that success.

Richard Lake

Copyright © 2002 by Mosby, Inc. All rights reserved.

Chapter 1

The Nursing Process and Drug Therapy

Choose the *best* answer for each of the following.

1. Which phase of the nursing process requires the nurse to establish a comprehensive baseline of data concerning a particular patient?
   a. Assessment
   b. Planning
   c. Implementation
   d. Evaluation

2. The nurse may revise or discontinue unrealistic goals during which phase of the nursing process?
   a. Assessment
   b. Planning
   c. Implementation
   d. Evaluation

3. Prescribed medications are prepared and administered during which phase of the nursing process?
   a. Assessment
   b. Planning
   c. Implementation
   d. Evaluation

4. Which of the following must occur for a goal statement to be patient-centered?
   a. Family input is essential.
   b. The patient must be involved in establishing the goal(s).
   c. The nurse must develop the goal(s).
   d. The physician must be involved in establishing the goal(s).

5. Which of the following is part of a complete medication history?
   a. Use of "street" drugs
   b. Current laboratory work
   c. Past history of surgeries
   d. Family history

Label each of the following as either objective data (O) or subjective data (S).

6. Below is a list of data gathered from an assessment of Ms. Biehle, a young woman visiting your clinic with what she describes as "maybe an ulcer."

   _____ Ms. Biehle tells you that she smokes a pack of cigarettes a day.

   _____ She is 5 feet 5 inches and weighs 135 pounds.

   _____ You find that her pulse and blood pressure are normal.

   _____ Her stool was tested for occult blood by a lab technician; the tests were negative.

   _____ Ms. Biehle says that she does not experience nausea, but she reports pain and heartburn, especially after eating popcorn—something she and her husband have always done while watching TV before bedtime.

   _____ She experiences occasional increases in stomach pain, "a feeling of heat" in her abdomen and chest at night when she lies down, and increased incidents of heartburn.

Copyright © 2002 by Mosby, Inc. All rights reserved.

CRITICAL THINKING AND APPLICATION

Answer the following questions on a separate sheet of paper.

7. Identify the "five rights" of drug administration, and specify ways to ensure that each of these rights is addressed.

8. The nursing process is an orderly and systematic method of identifying three components of a patient's health status and care. The three components are:

   a. _____

   b. _____

   c. _____

   Data is collected during the (d.) _____ phase of the nursing process.

   Data can be classified as (e.) _____ or (f.) _____.

   To formulate the nursing diagnosis, the nurse must first (g.) _____ the information collected.

   The planning phase includes identification of (h.) _____ and (i.) _____.

   The (j.) _____ phase consists of initiation and completion of the nursing care plan.

   The (k.) _____ phase is ongoing and includes monitoring the patient's response to medication and determining the status of goals.

9. Identify six ways to avoid medication errors. Explain what you should do if a medication error occurs.

Copyright © 2002 by Mosby, Inc. All rights reserved.

Chapter 2

Pharmacologic Principles

Choose the *best* answer for each of the following.

1. Another name for biotransformation of a drug is:
   a. absorption.
   b. dilution.
   c. excretion.
   d. metabolism.

2. Drug excretion occurs mainly from the:
   a. renal tubules and skin.
   b. skin and lungs.
   c. gastrointestinal tract and renal tubules.
   d. lungs and gastrointestinal tract.

3. Drugs that build up in the body systems as a result of excessive dosages, poor circulation, faulty metabolism, or inadequate excretion may result in:
   a. tolerance.
   b. cumulative effects.
   c. incompatibility.
   d. antagonistic effects.

4. Drug half-life is defined as the amount of time required by 50% of a drug to:
   a. be absorbed by the body.
   b. reach a therapeutic level.
   c. exert a response.
   d. be eliminated by the body.

5. Drugs given by which route are altered by the first-pass effect?
   a. Oral
   b. Sublingual
   c. Subcutaneous
   d. Intravenous

Match each field of study with its corresponding "job" description.

6. _____ Biopharmaceutics

7. _____ Pharmacokinetics

8. _____ Pharmacodynamics

9. _____ Pharmacogenetics

10. _____ Pharmacotherapeutics

11. _____ Pharmacognosy

12. _____ Chemotherapy

13. _____ Toxicology

14. _____ Teratogenesis

15. _____ Prophylactic therapy

a. Lisa is researching botanical and zoologic sources of drugs to treat MS; she is part of a university research team that is currently experimenting with varying the biochemical composition and therapeutic effects of several possible new drugs.

b. Jeffrey works for a pharmaceutical corporation. One of Lisa's teams' "new drugs" looks very promising, and Jeffrey's company is experimenting with dose forms for an investigational new drug. He is responsible for measuring the relationship between the physiochemical properties of the dosage form and the clinical therapeutic response.

c. Meiko examines case studies of patients with similar conditions and drug therapies in order to determine similarities in treatments and outcomes.

d. Hamische researches various poisons, particularly the detection and treatment of the effects of drugs and chemicals in certain mammals.

Copyright © 2002 by Mosby, Inc. All rights reserved.

e.   Steven represents a research firm that subcontracts with the FDA to observe and report on drug-induced congenital anomalies and the toxic effects drugs can have on the developing fetus.

f.   Diane and Phil have spent the last 3 years gathering family histories, legal cases, and current clinical data to discern possible genetic factors and their influence on individuals' responses to meperidine and related drugs.

g.   David works on a study that is gathering data on the empirical or rational application of two drugs for the treatment of rheumatoid arthritis.

h.   Michelle's research has taken her to Southeast Asia and Australia to participate in worldwide research on treatment of a neoplastic disease that occurs in higher percentages in those two regions.

i.   Leslie's laboratory monitors drug distribution rates between various body components, from absorption through excretion. Recently, her lab was able to suggest a positive change in the dosage regimen of an injectable drug, bringing her firm a prestigious award.

j.   Gregory's research unit recently recommended two new contraindications for a newly marketed drug after discovering previously unknown biochemical and physiologic interactions of this drug with another unrelated drug.

CRITICAL THINKING AND APPLICATION

Answer the following question on a separate sheet of paper.

16.   Mr. Cullen enters the trauma center in some distress. He is experiencing symptoms that demand quick absorption of a drug. If presented with the following choices, which route of administration would you use: subcutaneous or intramuscular? Mr. Cullen's physician asks you to further increase absorption—mechanically. How can you do this?

Copyright © 2002 by Mosby, Inc. All rights reserved.

Chapter 3

Lifespan Considerations

Choose the *best* answer for each of the following.

1. Which physiologic factor is most responsible for the differences in the pharmacokinetic and pharmacodynamic behavior of drugs in neonates and adults?
   a. The infant's stature
   b. The infant's smaller weight
   c. The immaturity of neonatal organs
   d. The adult's longer exposure to toxins

2. Which of the following drugs are more toxic in children?
   a. phenobarbital, morphine, and aspirin
   b. phenobarbital, morphine, and atropine
   c. theophylline, atropine, and digoxin
   d. morphine, atropine, and digoxin

3. The most common method of calculating doses for the pediatric patient is:
   a. based on total body water content.
   b. dependent on fat-to-lean mass ratio.
   c. based on height.
   d. based on weight.

4. The criteria for determining drug doses in the elderly should be based:
   a. more on age than on height or weight.
   b. more on weight than on age.
   c. on the total body water (TBW) content.
   d. on the glomerular filtration rate.

5. Which of the following statements is *not* true of the geriatric patient?
   a. Total body water content is increased as body composition changes.
   b. Gastric pH is less acidic because of reduced hydrochloric acid.
   c. Protein albumin binding sites are reduced because of decreased protein.
   d. Fat content is increased because of decreased lean body mass and altered TBW.

Match each pregnancy safety category with its corresponding description.

6. _____ Category A

7. _____ Category B

8. _____ Category C

9. _____ Category D

10. _____ Category X

a. Possible fetal risk in humans reported; however, potential benefit versus risk may, in selected cases, warrant the use of these drugs in pregnant women.

b. Studies indicate no risk to animal fetus; information in humans is not available.

c. Fetal abnormalities reported and positive evidence of fetal risk in humans is available from animal and/or human studies.

d. Studies indicate no risk to the fetus.

e. Adverse effects reported in animal fetus; information in humans is not available.

Copyright © 2002 by Mosby, Inc. All rights reserved.

CRITICAL THINKING AND APPLICATION

Answer the following questions on a separate sheet of paper.

11. You are a nurse at a community clinic frequented by a number of elderly patients. Mrs. Milner comes to your clinic, complaining of dizziness and nausea. As you take her medication history, she shows you her "pill box." Inside you see almost a dozen different pills, all to be taken at noon. How could this happen? How could she possibly need so many medications at the same time?

12. The physician confirms that Mrs. Milner's "new symptoms," as she refers to them, are a result of polypharmacy. She protests, telling you, "Honey, I've got news for the doctor. I've had to take lots of drugs at the same time all my life. It never bothered me before. Why would it now when I'm even more used to it?" Explain at least three physiologic changes that occur with aging and how these changes affect pharmacokinetics and pharmacodynamics.

Copyright © 2002 by Mosby, Inc. All rights reserved.

Chapter 4

Legal, Ethical, and Cultural Considerations

Choose the *best* answer for each of the following.

1. Which group of drugs would be classified as C-I, given "only with approved protocol?"
   a. codeine, cocaine, and meperidine
   b. heroin, LSD, and marijuana
   c. phenobarbital, chloral hydrate, and benzo-diazepines
   d. cough preparations and diarrhea control agents

2. When a health care provider is writing a prescription for a drug, which classification does *not* permit a refill to be marked on the prescription?
   a. C-II
   b. C-III
   c. C-IV
   d. C-V

3. The ethical principle of "do no harm" is known as:
   a. autonomy.
   b. beneficence.
   c. confidentiality.
   d. nonmaleficence.

4. Which legal act required drug manufacturers to establish the safety and efficacy of a new drug before its approval for use?
   a. Pure Food and Drug Act of 1906
   b. Food, Drug, and Cosmetic Act of 1938
   c. Kefauver-Harris Amendment of the 1938 Act
   d. Durham-Humphrey Amendment of the 1938 Act

5. Which definition correctly defines a "placebo?"
   a. An investigational drug used in a new drug study
   b. An inert substance that is not a drug
   c. A legend drug that requires a prescription
   d. A substance that is not approved as a drug but used as an herbal product

Match each investigational drug study phase with its corresponding description.

6. _____ Phase I

7. _____ Phase II

8. _____ Phase III

9. _____ Phase IV

a. A study using small numbers of volunteers who have the disease or disorder that the drug is meant to diagnose or treat. Subjects are monitored for drug efficacy and side effects.

b. Postmarketing studies used by drug companies to obtain further proof of the drug's therapeutic effects.

c. A study that involves a large number of patients at research centers to monitor for infrequent side effects and to identify any associated risks. Double-blind, placebo-controlled studies eliminate patient/researcher bias.

d. A study that uses small numbers of healthy volunteers, as opposed to volunteers afflicted with the target ailment, to determine dosage range and pharmacokinetics.

33

Copyright © 2002 by Mosby, Inc. All rights reserved.

Match each cultural group with its corresponding cultural practice.

10. _____ Asian

11. _____ Hispanic

12. _____ Native-American

13. _____ African-American

a. Some may seek a balance between the body and mind through the use of cold remedies or foods for "hot" illnesses—and vice versa.

b. Some may use folk medicine, protective bracelets, and laying on of hands.

c. Some believe that opposing forces of negative and positive energies lead to illness or health, depending on which force is in balance.

d. Some believe in the balance between the body, mind, and environment to maintain health and harmony with nature.

CRITICAL THINKING AND APPLICATION

Answer the following questions on a separate sheet of paper.

14. Identify a cultural group in your area, and explore the health belief practices for that group.

   a. Are there any barriers to adequate health care?

   b. What is the attitude toward Western medicines and health treatments?

   c. What questions should you ask in your cultural assessment?

Copyright © 2002 by Mosby, Inc. All rights reserved.

Chapter 5

Patient Education and Drug Therapy

CRITICAL THINKING AND APPLICATION

Answer the following questions on a separate sheet of paper.

1. You are to present information regarding antihypertensive drug therapy to two patients. One patient is 40 years old; the other is 78. Describe the differences in interventions you would use in your teaching strategies related to possible alterations in thought processes and sensory-perceptual status in these two patients.

2. You are to present information to a young mother on how to help her 8-year-old child use a metered-dose inhaler. Neither the mother nor her child speaks English. Discuss strategies to use while developing a teaching plan for them.

3. Your patient has been taking oral hypoglycemics for 1 month, and her blood glucose readings are still very high. On assessment, you discover a possible reason for these high readings. Develop a nursing diagnosis for this patient based on the following:

   a. The patient says that no one has ever told her about needed dietary restrictions.

   b. The patient tells you that she takes the medication only when she remembers it.

4. For each of the following medications, develop a measurable goal and specific outcome criteria related to teaching a patient about the medication therapy. Use later chapters in the textbook for reference.

   a. Oral contraceptives

   b. Diuretic therapy, furosemide

   c. digoxin

   d. Transdermal nitroglycerin patches

   e. indomethacin

5. Develop a patient teaching plan for a 55-year-old patient who will be discharged on warfarin therapy. Refer to the appropriate chapter in the text for information. Include the following:

   a. Assessment of the objective and subjective data that would be needed

   b. The nursing diagnosis

   c. Planning—including a measurable goal and outcome criteria

   d. Implementation—specific educational strategies

   e. Evaluation—how you would validate that learning had occurred

Copyright © 2002 by Mosby, Inc. All rights reserved.

Chapter 6

Over-the-Counter Drugs and Herbal Remedies

CRITICAL THINKING CROSSWORD

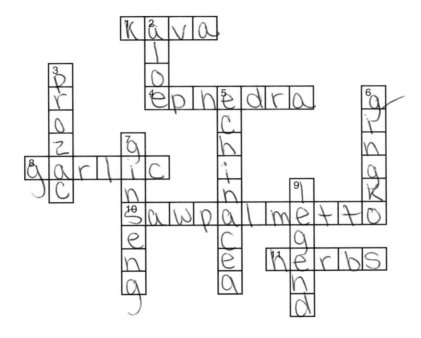

Across

1. Used to relieve anxiety, stress, and restlessness; may cause skin discoloration.
4. Also known as "herbal fen-fen."
8. Used for its antiplatelet activity.
10. Used for benign prostatic hypertrophy.
11. Plants used for healing purposes are known as _____.

Down

2. Topical application of this plant has been used to help aid wound healing.
3. St. John's wort is used for depression and is known as "herbal _____."
5. Herbs most commonly used to treat colds and chronic infections of the respiratory and urinary tract.
6. An herb known to worsen GI disorders and bleeding tendencies; interacts with NSAIDs and tricyclic antidepressants.
7. Dried roots used as a tonic for invigoration, fortification, and concentration.
9. Drugs that require a prescription for purchase are _____ drugs.

Copyright © 2002 by Mosby, Inc. All rights reserved.

Choose the *best* answer for each of the following.

1. Classifications of drugs commonly used as over-the-counter remedies include all of the following *except*:
   a. NSAIDs.
   b. cold remedies.
   c. antibiotics.
   d. nicotine smoking deterrent systems.

2. Patients who take NSAIDs should be taught to:
   a. take the medication with food to decrease GI symptoms.
   b. take the medication on an empty stomach to improve absorption.
   c. expect immediate results from therapy.
   d. crush or break open caplets and capsules for ease of swallowing.

3. Patients taking an H_2 antagonist such as cimetidine should remember to take it:
   a. with an antacid to improve relief.
   b. 1 hour before or after antacids.
   c. only if spicy foods are eaten.
   d. on an empty stomach.

4. An herb commonly used for external treatment of insect bites and minor burns is:
   a. feverfew.
   b. yarrow.
   c. aloe vera.
   d. valerian.

5. Advantages of over-the-counter remedies include which of the following?
   a. Third-party health insurance payers usually cover the costs.
   b. Patients can feel better faster when self-medicating.
   c. There are fewer drug interactions.
   d. Patients can self-treat minor ailments and reduce physician visits.

6. Patients taking OTC cromolyn need to be reminded that:
   a. this medication is used for acute bronchospams.
   b. this medication is safe for use while pregnant.
   c. this medication reduces the need to check peak flow rates.
   d. true therapeutic effects may not be seen for 4 weeks.

CRITICAL THINKING AND APPLICATION

Answer the following question on a separate sheet of paper.

7. Which herbal products and OTC medications discussed in this chapter interact with anticoagulants?

Copyright © 2002 by Mosby, Inc. All rights reserved.

Chapter 7

Substance Abuse

Match each drug with its corresponding description.

1. _____ cocaine

2. _____ methamphetamine

3. _____ phenobarbital

4. _____ heroin

5. _____ disulfiram

6. _____ nicotine

7. _____ naltrexone

8. _____ Zyban

9. _____ opium

10. _____ "roofies"

a. A nicotine-free treatment for nicotine dependence.

b. Known as the "date rape" drug.

c. The source plant for heroin.

d. The addictive chemical in tobacco products.

e. An opioid that is injected by "mainlining" or "skin-popping."

f. Used for withdrawal from barbiturates.

g. Used to deter the use of alcohol during alcohol abuse treatment.

h. A stimulant that is either "snorted" through the nasal passages or injected intravenously.

i. A stimulant that is popular at "raves" with college-age students.

j. An opioid antagonist used for opioid abuse/dependence.

Choose the _best_ answer for each of the following.

11. A patient who has been on Antabuse (disulfiram) therapy for 3 months has been off the therapy for 2 days. He decides to go out with friends to have a beer. What effects may he experience?
    a. No ill effects
    b. Diarrhea
    c. Vomiting
    d. Euphoria

12. The most common drug effects leading to abuse of opioids include:
    a. hallucinations.
    b. sleep.
    c. stimulation.
    d. relaxation and euphoria.

13. All of the following medications may be used for opioid withdrawal _except_:
    a. disulfiram (Antabuse).
    b. clonidine (Catapres).
    c. methadone.
    d. naltrexone (ReVia).

14. The combination of benzodiazepines with ethanol or barbiturates may lead to death by:
    a. cardiac dysrhythmia.
    b. convulsions.
    c. respiratory arrest.
    d. stroke.

15. Chronic excessive ingestion of ethanol is directly associated with the development of disorders such as:
    a. lung cancer.
    b. Korsakoff's psychosis.
    c. ulcerative colitis.
    d. chronic renal failure.

39

Copyright © 2002 by Mosby, Inc. All rights reserved.

CRITICAL THINKING AND APPLICATION

Answer the following question on a separate sheet of paper.

16. Describe how nicotine is used to help withdrawal from nicotine use. How is bupropion (Zyban) used in smoking cessation programs?

Copyright © 2002 by Mosby, Inc. All rights reserved.

Chapter 8

Photo Atlas of Drug Administration

Choose the *best* answer for each of the following.

1. To expel air bubbles after drawing fluid from an ampule, remove the needle, hold the syringe with the needle pointing up, and do which of the following?
   a. Draw back slightly on the plunger, tap the side of the syringe to cause bubbles to rise toward the needle, and push the plunger upward to eject air.
   b. Tap the side of the syringe to cause bubbles to rise toward the needle, draw back slightly on the plunger, and push the plunger upward to eject air.
   c. Tap the side of the syringe to cause bubbles to rise toward the needle, draw back slightly on the plunger, push the plunger upward to eject air, and eject a small amount of fluid.
   d. Draw back slightly on the plunger, tap the side of the syringe to cause bubbles to rise toward the needle, and push the plunger upward to eject air; do not eject fluid.

2. For intradermal injections:
   a. massage the site lightly.
   b. have the patient massage the site until the pain diminishes.
   c. do not massage the site.
   d. apply heat to the site.

3. When administering medication by IV push, occlude the IV line by:
   a. pinching the tubing just above the injection port.
   b. pinching the tubing at least 2 inches above the injection port.
   c. folding the tubing just above the injection port.
   d. no means; it is not necessary to occlude the tubing.

4. When more than one medication is to be added to a solution:
   a. use an equal volume of each.
   b. assess them for drug compatibility.
   c. always add them at least 1 hour apart.
   d. use the same needle for both medications.

5. When administering oral medications:
   a. crush all medications and spoon them into the mouth for patients who are unable to hold them.
   b. allow powdered medications and liquids to sit at least 1 minute after mixing them together.
   c. stay with the patient until each medication has been swallowed.
   d. give all medications with meals to facilitate absorption.

6. After administering eardrops:
   a. press a cotton ball firmly into the ear.
   b. have the patient sit up and tilt the head for 2 to 3 minutes.
   c. gently massage the tragus of the ear.
   d. have the patient remain in the side-lying position for 15 minutes.

7. To administer nasal drops for the frontal or maxillary sinus:
   a. tilt the patient's head backward and facing toward the left side.
   b. tilt the patient's head back over the edge of the bed with the head turned toward the side treated.
   c. place a pillow under the patient's shoulders and tilt the head back.
   d. tilt the patient's head to the side opposite the side treated.

8. With NG tubes:
   a. always allow any fluid to flow via gravity.
   b. use gentle but consistent pressure when forcing the fluid into the tube.
   c. shake the tube gently to facilitate the movement of fluid in the tube.
   d. confirm placement of the tube after the medication is given.

41

Copyright © 2002 by Mosby, Inc. All rights reserved.

9. Z-track intramuscular injections are indicated in which of the following situations?
   a. When there is insufficient muscle mass in the landmarked area
   b. Whenever massaging the area after medication administration is contraindicated
   c. With medications that are known to be irritating, painful, and/or staining to tissues
   d. With any injection that is given into the ventrogluteal muscle

10. Sublingual medications have the advantage of being:
    a. immediately absorbed.
    b. excreted rapidly.
    c. metabolized minimally.
    d. distributed equally.

11. The dosage of a Compazine rectal suppository is twice what has actually been ordered. Your most appropriate intervention would be to:
    a. cut the suppository in half.
    b. call the doctor for clarification.
    c. administer another type of suppository.
    d. instruct the patient to retain the suppository for only 5 minutes.

12. Which of the following is a contraindication for the administration of rectal suppositories?
    a. Vomiting
    b. Fever
    c. Constipation
    d. Hemorrhoids

13. Transdermal (skin) administration of medications is enhanced when the skin is:
    a. intact.
    b. macerated.
    c. atrophied.
    d. moist.

14. Which of the following is important when teaching the patient about the instillation of nasal drops?
    a. Clear the nasal passages by blowing the nose gently before administering the medication.
    b. Clear the nasal passages by blowing the nose gently after administering the medication.
    c. Sit in a semi-Fowler's position for 5 minutes after the instillation of medications.
    d. Place the nose dropper approximately ½ inch into the nostril when instilling drops.

15. Which of the following is *not* true regarding the administration of ophthalmic medications?
    a. Have the patient look upward while instilling the medication.
    b. Instill the prescribed number of drops into the conjunctival sac.
    c. Apply gentle pressure to the patient's nasolacrimal duct for 30 to 60 seconds after instilling the drops.
    d. Apply ointment to the conjunctival sac starting at the outer canthus and working toward the inner canthus.

CRITICAL THINKING AND APPLICATION

Answer the following questions on a separate sheet of paper.

16. Describe how you assess injection sites for each of the following: a. SC injections; b. IM injections; c. ID injections.

17. Describe the proper technique of needle insertion for each of the following: a. SC injections; b. IM injections; c. ID injections.

18. You are administering an IM injection to your patient. After the needle enters the site, you grasp the lower end of the syringe barrel with your nondominant hand and slowly pull back on the plunger to aspirate the drug. Blood appears in the syringe. What do you do?

19. You are preparing a liquid medication for a patient. How does the usual procedure change when the volume of medication required is less than 10 ml?

Copyright © 2002 by Mosby, Inc. All rights reserved.

Chapter 9

Analgesic Agents

CRITICAL THINKING CROSSWORD

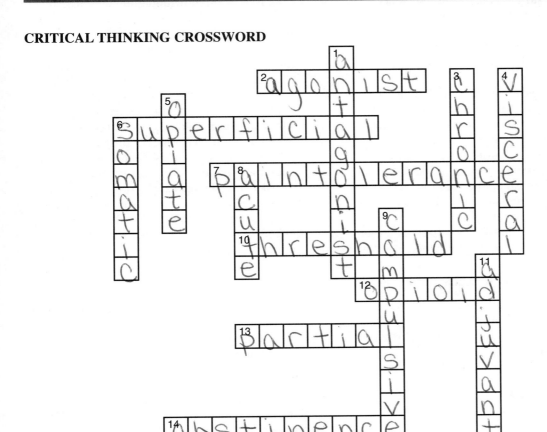

Across

2. Any drug that binds to a receptor and causes a response has _____ properties.
6. Mrs. G suffers from psoriasis, a very uncomfortable skin disorder. Mrs. G comes in rubbing her hands and complaining of _____ pain.
7. Mr. R, from 12 Across, is recovering. He requires continued pain management but is able to take less powerful doses of medication now. Every day he tells you that he finds he can do "more and more normal things, even though there is still some pain there." Mr. R is describing his level of _____ (two words).
10. Ms. L was in an accident with a resultant leg injury. In assessing the level of stimulus applied to her toe that results in a perception of pain, you are testing her pain _____.

12. Mr. R is brought to the emergency room in tremendous pain. The ER team recognizes the need to immediately bring the pain under some control to make assessment, diagnosis, and treatment more manageable. After assessing that it is not contraindicated, the attending physician initiates administration of a very strong and addicting pain reliever. This is no doubt a(n) _____ analgesic.
13. Ms. T is taking a drug that binds to part of a receptor and causes effects that are less pronounced than those of a pure agonist. She is taking a _____ agonist.
14. Mr. Y is suffering the effects of having withdrawn from an opioid analgesic; he had become physically dependent on the drug, and now that he no longer has access to it, he is suffering opioid _____ syndrome.

Copyright © 2002 by Mosby, Inc. All rights reserved.

Down

1. Mr. D's drug binds to a receptor but causes the opposite effect as the type of drug discussed in 13 Across. He is taking a drug with _____ properties.
3. Mrs. H has suffered back pain "for years." She says that it is worse in the late afternoon and at night, but that "really, even when it lessens somewhat, it is there all the time in some form." Mrs. H is seeking relief from _____ pain.
4. Mr. E paces the floor all night, holding his side. The pain is so severe that he is sick to his stomach. His wife brings him into the emergency room, where it is quickly discerned that Mr. E has a kidney stone. The type of pain he has been experiencing is _____ pain.
5. Mr. K is put on an opioid pain reliever; its main active ingredient is opium, making this drug a(n) _____ analgesic.
6. Mr. J has injured himself in a friendly basketball game with his peers after work. His wife brings him to the urgent care center several hours later because of the pain. Mr. J. is probably experiencing _____ pain.
8. Mrs. M regularly experiences sudden, severe headaches that leave her incapacitated. However, when she takes her prescription medication, it takes effect within minutes and resolves fairly quickly. Mrs. M's headaches fall in the realm of _____ pain.
9. Mr. C has entered a treatment center to help him overcome a psychologic dependence on a cocaine derivative. What he is seeking help for is a _____ use of this drug, characterized by a continuous craving that is not pain-related.
11. Mr. V is already taking an opioid pain reliever. When his pain increases, the drug is not as effective. He is given a second opioid agent in addition to the first drug. "Two pain killers?" he asks you. "Is that safe?" You explain that the second drug is not a primary analgesic but has properties that will add to the analgesic effects of the opioid. It is being used, then, as a(n) _____ agent.

Choose the *best* answer for each of the following.

1. Mr. Verdi recently competed in a marathon. After running 16 miles, he had to drop out because of severe muscle spasms. This type of pain is classified as:
   a. chronic pain.
   b. somatic pain.
   c. visceral pain.
   d. superficial pain.

2. A 23-year-old has been taken to the emergency room for a suspected overdose of morphine tablets. Which agent may be used to treat this overdose?
   a. Demerol
   b. Naprosyn
   c. aspirin
   d. Narcan

3. An analgesic is given to:
   a. produce sleep.
   b. relieve nausea.
   c. relieve pain.
   d. reduce the level of consciousness prior to surgery.

4. Moderate-to-severe pain is best treated with:
   a. acetaminophen.
   b. naloxone.
   c. propoxyphene.
   d. morphine sulfate.

5. Premedication assessments prior to administering an opiate agonist include all of the following *except*:
   a. rating the level of pain on a scale.
   b. prior analgesic use (time, type, amount, and effectiveness).
   c. allergies.
   d. blood clotting times.

Copyright © 2002 by Mosby, Inc. All rights reserved.

Match each type of pain with its corresponding description.

6. _g_ Acute pain

7. _f_ Chronic pain

8. _i_ Somatic pain

9. _h_ Visceral pain

10. _d_ Superficial pain

11. _b_ Vascular pain

12. _j_ Neuropathic pain

13. _c_ Phantom pain

14. _a_ Psychogenic pain

15. _e_ Central pain

a. Pain that is due to psychologic factors, not physical conditions or disorders.

b. Pain that is thought to account for most migraine headaches.

c. Pain that occurs in a body part that has been removed.

d. Pain that originates from the skin or mucous membranes.

e. Pain that occurs with tumors, trauma, or inflammation of the brain.

f. Persistent or recurring pain that is often difficult to treat.

g. Pain that is sudden in onset and usually subsides when treated.

h. Pain that originates from the organs or smooth muscles.

i. Pain that originates from the skeletal muscles, ligaments, or joints.

j. Pain that results from injury or damage to the peripheral nerve fibers.

Copyright © 2002 by Mosby, Inc. All rights reserved.

Chapter 10

General and Local Anesthetics

CRITICAL THINKING CROSSWORD

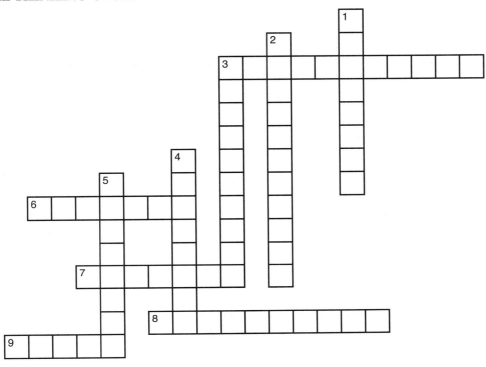

Across

3. A commonly used long-acting, nondepolariz-ing NMBA.
6. Anesthetic agents that have global effects, including loss of consciousness and deep mus-cle relaxation.
7. A class of anesthetics applied directly to the skin and mucous membranes.
8. Agents used in combination with anesthetic agents to control the side effects of anesthetics.
9. Anesthetic agents that render a specific portion of the body insensitive to pain without affect-ing consciousness.

Down

1. An antidote for overdose of succinylcholine chloride.
2. A broad term for agents that depress the CNS.
3. Anesthetics administered directly into the CNS by various spinal injection techniques.
4. The practice of using combinations of drugs to produce anesthesia rather than using a single agent.
5. Another name for 9 Across.

Copyright © 2002 by Mosby, Inc. All rights reserved.

Choose the *best* answer for each of the following.

1. Adjunctive agents used with anesthesia include all the following *except*:
   a. sedative-hypnotics.
   b. opioid analgesics.
   c. anticholinergics.
   d. inhaled gas.

2. Lidocaine is frequently used for:
   a. spinal anesthesia.
   b. local anesthesia.
   c. intravenous anesthesia.
   d. general anesthesia.

3. Possible complications as a result of NMBA use include:
   a. induction of apnea.
   b. headache.
   c. bradycardia.
   d. hypertension.

4. To decrease the possibility of a headache after spinal anesthesia, you should instruct the patient to:
   a. sit in high-Fowler's position.
   b. lie flat in bed.
   c. limit fluids.
   d. engage in activity.

5. Local anesthesia is indicated for all the following *except*:
   a. spinal anesthesia.
   b. suturing a skin laceration.
   c. long-duration surgery.
   d. diagnostic procedures.

6. A sudden elevation in body temperature in a patient who has just returned from surgery may indicate:
   a. a normal temperature change after surgery.
   b. malignant hypertension.
   c. malignant hyperthermia.
   d. fever.

CRITICAL THINKING AND APPLICATION

Answer the following questions on a separate sheet of paper.

7. Henry is a student nurse who has assisted the anesthetist in surgery on prior occasions. Today, however, he is nervous because it is a child who will undergo general anesthesia. Why might this make Henry more nervous than usual?

8. Mr. Smith is being administered a neuromuscular blocking agent while receiving mechanical ventilation. What is important to remember when working with him while he is on this therapy?

Copyright © 2002 by Mosby, Inc. All rights reserved.

Chapter 11

Central Nervous System Depressants and Muscle Relaxants

Choose the *best* answer for each of the following.

1. A hypnotic is an agent that:
   - (a.) produces sleep.
   - b. slows the destruction of dopamine.
   - c. prevents nausea and vomiting.
   - d. relaxes the patient.

2. A patient who has been taking a benzodiazepine for 5 weeks is told by his physician that he wants him to stop using the medication. The best way to discontinue the medication is to:
   - a. stop taking the drug immediately.
   - (b.) plan a gradual reduction in dosage.
   - c. overlap the initial medication with another agent.
   - d. take the medication every other day for weeks.

3. Which type of barbiturate is used as an anesthetic for short surgical procedures?
   - (a.) Ultrashort
   - b. Short
   - c. Intermediate
   - d. Long

4. The cause of death from an overdose of barbiturates is:
   - a. tachycardia.
   - b. hypertension.
   - c. dyspnea.
   - (d.) respiratory arrest.

5. Musculoskeletal relaxants are most effective when used in conjunction with:
   - a. benzodiazepines.
   - b. bed rest.
   - (c.) physical therapy.
   - d. aspirin.

CRITICAL THINKING AND APPLICATION

Answer the following questions on a separate sheet of paper.

6. A 19-year-old college freshman is brought into the emergency room with a suspected barbiturate overdose. What symptoms would you expect to see? How is overdose treated?

7. Jackie is taking benzodiazepines to treat her insomnia. Today she visits your clinic and states that she is going to Europe for 2 months and wants a prescription that will allow her to take enough medication along for her entire stay. The physician declines. She is a little insulted and asks you why he refused her request. "Does he think I'm an addict or suicidal or something?"

8. Mrs. Alexander, who is 81 years of age, weighs significantly more than her 47-year-old daughter; yet she is given a lower dose of medication for insomnia of a similar degree. Why? Is this a dose calculation error?

Copyright © 2002 by Mosby, Inc. All rights reserved.

9. You have been asked to take a patient history for William, who will be given a benzodiazepine.

   a. What conditions or disorders should you ask about?

   b. What drug intake should you be most concerned about?

   c. What if William were an infant? A great-grandfather? Would this additional information matter? Why or why not?

10. Mr. Palmer is recovering from an automobile accident and has received a prescription for cyclobenzaprine for painful muscle spasms.

    a. What patient teaching should he receive about this medication?

    b. What other measures should be included with this drug therapy?

11. Define tachyphylaxis and name one drug that can cause it. Is it an advantage or disadvantage? Why?

Copyright © 2002 by Mosby, Inc. All rights reserved.

Chapter 12

Antiepileptic Agents

CRITICAL THINKING CROSSWORD

Across

2. Status epilepticus is considered a medical _____.
6. A type of epilepsy with an unknown cause.
10. A potentially fatal side effect of valproic acid.
11. A brief episode of abnormal electrical activity.
12. Intravenously administered AEDs should be delivered this way to avoid serious side effects.

Down

1. A type of epilepsy with a distinct cause.
3. A spasmodic contraction of involuntary muscles.
4. Considered first-line agents in the treatment of status epilepticus.
5. Another term for 6 Across.
6. A barbiturate used primarily to control tonic-clonic and partial seizures.
7. The metabolic process that occurs when a drug increases its own metabolism over time, leading to lower-than-expected drug concentrations.
8. Chronic, recurrent pattern of seizures.
9. Therapeutic levels for this drug are 5 to 20 µg/dl, and long-term use can cause gingival hyperplasia.

Copyright © 2002 by Mosby, Inc. All rights reserved.

Choose the *best* answer for each of the following.

1. Janie has seizures characterized by temporary lapses in consciousness that last only a few seconds. Her teachers have said that she "daydreams too much." These types of seizures are:
   a. simple seizures.
   b. complex seizures.
   c. partial seizures.
   d. generalized seizures.

2. Which condition is a life-threatening emergency in which patients typically do not regain consciousness?
   a. Status epilepticus
   b. Tonic-clonic convulsions
   c. Epilepsy
   d. Primary epilepsy

3. Which of the following is *not* true about intravenous infusion of phenytoin?
   a. It should be injected quickly.
   b. It should be injected slowly.
   c. It should be followed by an injection of sterile saline.
   d. Continuous infusion should be avoided.

4. Which of the following is a possible side/adverse effect of phenobarbital therapy?
   a. Constipation
   b. Gingival hyperplasia
   c. Drowsiness
   d. Dysrhythmias

5. Which drug would be used for the treatment of status epilepticus?
   a. phenobarbital
   b. diazepam
   c. valproic acid
   d. phenytoin

CRITICAL THINKING AND APPLICATION

Answer the following questions on a separate sheet of paper.

6. What is meant by autoinduction in a drug? Identify at least one AED that undergoes autoinduction.

7. Jeremy, an 8-year-old, has resisted his oral doses of topiramate, which has made compliance difficult. His mother calls and says that she has found a way to get him to take it: she crushes it and sprinkles it on gelatin. She is delighted. What is your response?

Copyright © 2002 by Mosby, Inc. All rights reserved.

Chapter 13

Antiparkinsonian Agents

Choose the *best* answer for each of the following.

1. Your patient with Parkinson's disease has difficulty performing voluntary movements. This is known as:
   a. akinesia.
   b. dyskinesia.
   c. chorea.
   d. dystonia.

2. Which drug may be used early in the treatment of Parkinson's disease but eventually loses effectiveness and must be replaced by another agent?
   a. amantadine
   b. levodopa
   c. selegiline
   d. tolcapone

3. Mr. Ford, who is taking levodopa for Parkinson's disease, wants to take a vitamin supplement. What should he be told?
   a. Be sure to take a supplement that provides all vitamins and minerals.
   b. Be sure to take a supplement twice a day to ensure enough nutrients.
   c. Avoid supplements that contain vitamin B_6 (pyridoxine).
   d. Do not take more than the recommended amount of calcium with this medication.

4. A patient who is newly diagnosed with Parkinson's disease and beginning medication therapy asks the nurse, "How soon will improvement occur?" The nurse's best response is:
   a. "That varies from patient to patient."
   b. "You should discuss that with your physician."
   c. "You should notice a difference in a few days."
   d. "It may take several weeks before you notice any degree of improvement."

5. Anticholinergic agents administered during treatment of Parkinson's disease are given to control or minimize all the following symptoms *except*:
   a. drooling.
   b. constipation.
   c. muscle rigidity.
   d. tremors.

CRITICAL THINKING AND APPLICATION

Answer the following questions on a separate sheet of paper.

6. Mr. Hicks is about to have levodopa added to his carbidopa treatment regimen.

   a. Why must dopamine be administered in the form of levodopa?

   b. What problems are avoided when carbidopa is given with levodopa?

   c. Why?

7. Mrs. Reynolds, a 35-year-old new mother, has experienced slowing movements, cogwheel rigidity, and pill-rolling tremor. Sadly, she has been diagnosed with Parkinson's disease, a somewhat rare phenomenon in someone her age. In addition to the usual history questions, what must you ask in anticipation of dopaminergic therapy in Mrs. Reynold's specific situation?

Copyright © 2002 by Mosby, Inc. All rights reserved.

8. Jane, age 45, is taking benztropine in addition to a dopaminergic agent for Parkinson's disease. Her 76-year-old neighbor comments that he cannot take benztropine because it is too risky for his heart and kidneys. Jane calls and asks why this isn't a concern in her case. What do you say?

Copyright © 2002 by Mosby, Inc. All rights reserved.

Chapter 14

Psychotherapeutic Agents

Match each term with its corresponding definition or description.

1. _____ sertraline

2. _____ Barbiturates

3. _____ Tricyclics

4. _____ Psychosis

5. _____ Mania

6. _____ diazepam

7. _____ amitriptyline

8. _____ nifedipine

9. _____ Benzodiazepines

10. _____ lithium

11. _____ Anxiety

12. _____ Affective disorders

13. _____ Depression

14. _____ phenelzine

15. _____ Bipolar affective disorder

a. The unpleasant state of mind in which unreal or imagined dangers are anticipated.

b. A state characterized by an expansive, emotional state (including symptoms of extreme excitement and elation) and hyperactivity.

c. A group of psychotropic agents prescribed to alleviate anxiety.

d. Emotional disorders characterized by changes in mood.

e. A major psychologic disorder characterized by episodes of mania, depression, or mixed mood.

f. Classified as a monoamine oxidase inhibitor.

g. One of the earliest drug classes used to treat anxiety.

h. Antidepressant agents that block reuptake of amine neuro transmitters.

i. An abnormal emotional state characterized by exaggerated feelings of sadness, melancholy, and worthlessness out of proportion to reality.

j. The most frequently prescribed benzodiazepine.

k. The most widely used tricyclic antidepressant.

l. Patients on MAOIs should have this drug available in case of inadvertent tyramine ingestion.

m. A second-generation antidepressant.

n. The drug of choice for mania.

o. A term used to describe a major emotional disorder that impairs the mental function of the affected individual to the extent that the individual cannot participate in everyday life.

Copyright © 2002 by Mosby, Inc. All rights reserved.

Choose the *best* answer for each of the following.

16. Patients taking the newer antipsychotic agents such as quetiapine (Seroquel) should be cautioned about which problem when beginning this therapy?
    a. Mood swings
    b. Diarrhea
    c. Postural hypotension
    d. Anorexia

17. When giving hydroxyzine intramuscularly, what measures should be taken?
    a. Use the Z-track method.
    b. Use a large-gauge needle.
    c. Apply an ice-pack to the site for 20 minutes.
    d. Divide the dose into two injections.

18. Leslie's husband Frank has been started on antidepressant therapy. She asks you, "How long will it take for him to feel better?" Your response should be:
    a. "Well, depression rarely responds to medication therapy."
    b. "He should be feeling better in a few days."
    c. "It may take 4 to 6 weeks before you see an improvement."
    d. "You may not see any effects for several months."

19. Extrapyramidal effects of drugs include all of the following *except*:
    a. spasmodic movement of limbs and the inability to sit still.
    b. elation and a sense of well-being.
    c. parkinsonian-like symptoms (such as a mask-like facial expression).
    d. involuntary motor restlessness.

20. The patient on MAOI therapy must be taught to avoid tyramine-containing foods in order to prevent which medical emergency?
    a. Gastric hemorrhage
    b. Toxic shock
    c. Cardiac arrest
    d. Severe hypertensive crisis

CRITICAL THINKING AND APPLICATION

Answer the following questions on a separate sheet of paper.

21. Carl, a 26-year-old unemployed electrician, is brought to the ER by his sister. He is extremely drowsy and confused, his breathing is slow and shallow, and he smells strongly of whiskey. The sister tells you that Carl has been seeing a psychiatrist for his "anxiety."

    a. What do you suspect might be wrong with Carl?

    b. How will he likely be treated?

22. Mr. Delvecchio, a 49-year-old restaurant owner, has been prescribed Nardil. After the physician leaves the room, but before you have a chance to discuss Mr. Delvecchio's medication regimen with him, he turns to his wife and says, "I'm sure this medicine will work. Let's have a bottle of wine tonight to celebrate."

    a. What should you say?

    b. A few weeks later, Mr. Delvecchio is brought to the ER with a severe headache, stiff neck, sweating, and elevated blood pressure. His wife says his symptoms started a few minutes after they ate at their restaurant. What is wrong with Mr. Delvecchio, and what probably caused it?

    c. What additional medication do you expect will be prescribed for Mr. Delvecchio?

23. Beth has been diagnosed with depression. She also has a history of anorexia and asthma. Why might the physician prescribe a second-generation antidepressant instead of a first-generation antidepressant?

Copyright © 2002 by Mosby, Inc. All rights reserved.

Chapter 15

Central Nervous System Stimulant Agents

Choose the *best* answer for each of the following.

1. Doxapram is commonly used to:
   a. control increased respiration effects of other drugs.
   b. treat respiratory insufficiency associated with COPD.
   c. treat postoperative elevated respiratory excitation.
   d. stimulate respirations in patients with head injury.

2. Which is *not* a contraindication of doxapram?
   a. Epilepsy
   b. Severe hypertension
   c. Cerebrovascular accident
   d. Narrow-angle glaucoma

3. CNS stimulants have which effect on the respiratory system?
   a. Relaxation of bronchial smooth muscle
   b. Decreased respiration
   c. Constriction of pulmonary arteries
   d. Decreased fatigue

4. Serotonin agonists are newer CNS stimulants used to treat:
   a. ADHD.
   b. hypertension.
   c. migraine headaches.
   d. narcolepsy.

5. Orlistat (Xenical) is a new anorexiant used to treat:
   a. anorexia.
   b. malnutrition.
   c. narcolepsy.
   d. obesity.

CRITICAL THINKING AND APPLICATION

Answer the following questions on a separate sheet of paper.

6. Stacey King, age 35, reports that she falls asleep unexpectedly at work, in class, and even while singing in her city's madrigal choir.

   a. What is wrong with Stacey?

   b. What might be the drug of choice for Stacey?

   c. Describe the therapeutic effects of such drugs.

   d. Draw up a patient teaching plan for Stacey. Offer guidelines for (1) dosage alterations and (2) substances she might be wise to avoid.

7. Five-year-old Jeffrey is taking methylphenidate for ADHD. What specific precautions must be taken with children who are taking this drug? Why?

Copyright © 2002 by Mosby, Inc. All rights reserved.

Chapter 16

Adrenergic Agents

Choose the *best* answer for each of the following.

1. Another name for adrenergic drugs is:
   a. anticholinergic agents.
   b. parasympathetic agents.
   c. central nervous system agents.
   d. sympathomimetic agents.

2. Adrenergic drugs produce which of the following effects?
   a. Urinary retention
   b. Bronchial constriction
   c. Increased heart rate and contractility
   d. Decreased intestinal motility

3. Adrenergic drugs may be used for all the following conditions *except*:
   a. asthma.
   b. glaucoma.
   c. nasal congestion.
   d. seizures.

4. Tina has just been stung by a bee, and she is panicking because she is allergic to bees. Her bee-sting kit would most likely contain:
   a. epinephrine.
   b. methylphenidate HCl.
   c. dopamine.
   d. norepinephrine.

5. Sandra, age 13, was diagnosed with asthma 2 years ago. Today her physician wants to start salmeterol. Which of the following is important to remember when teaching Sandra and her parents about this drug?
   a. It should be taken at the first sign of bronchospasms.
   b. The dosage is two puffs every 4 hours or any time needed for asthma attacks.
   c. It is not to be used for relief of acute symptoms; it is intended for long-term maintenance.
   d. If a steroid inhaler is also prescribed, the steroid should be taken first.

CRITICAL THINKING AND APPLICATION

Answer the following questions on a separate sheet of paper.

6. Three-year-old Kyle is taking pseudoephedrine drops as a nasal decongestant.

   a. What actions should promote easier nasal breathing for Kyle?

   b. Kyle's mother comes back to the clinic and complains that after a week his congestion is worse, not better. What possible explanation can you offer?

7. Mr. Dickens, a patient in the oncology ward, develops septic shock and is prescribed dopamine. However, something tells you that you should double-check Mr. Dickens' eligibility for this drug. What makes you think this?

8. Mr. Ganaden and Mr. Cowan are both on dopamine infusions. Mr. Ganaden's infusion is a low infusion rate, and Mr. Cowan's is a high infusion rate. Can you explain why these infusion rates might be different?

9. Mrs. Brooks is receiving epinephrine for emergent treatment of a cardiac rhythm problem. The physician mentions that he might try isoproterenol next. What would you say about this?

Copyright © 2002 by Mosby, Inc. All rights reserved.

Chapter 17

Adrenergic-Blocking Agents

Choose the *best* answer for each of the following.

1. Adrenergic blockade at the alpha-adrenergic receptors leads to all the following *except*:
   a. vasodilation.
   b. increased blood pressure.
   c. decreased blood pressure.
   d. constriction of the pupil.

2. Which agent is useful for reversing the potent vasoconstriction that occurs when vasopressors leak out of the blood vessel into the surrounding tissue?
   a. phentolamine
   b. prazosin
   c. ergotamine
   d. metoprolol

3. Liz suffers from migraine headaches. Her physician is considering treatment with ergotamine tartrate sublingual tablets. Which of the following is a contraindication?
   a. Asthma
   b. GERD
   c. Pregnancy
   d. Hypotension

4. Mr. Smith has been given prazosin as treatment for benign prostatic hypertrophy. What is important to include when teaching him about the effects of this medication?
   a. Watch for weight loss of 2 pounds within 2 weeks.
   b. Avoid caffeine.
   c. Take extra supplements of calcium.
   d. Change position slowly to avoid orthostatic changes.

5. Cheri has been taking propranolol for almost 6 months. When she comes in for a follow-up visit, she tells you that she wants to stop taking her medicine. In fact, you find out that she has not had any medication for over 24 hours. Is this a concern?
   a. No; there are no ill effects if this medication is stopped.
   b. No; after this amount of time there should be minimal effects if she stops the medication.
   c. Yes; she will probably experience rebound hypotension.
   d. Yes; sudden withdrawal of the drug may cause underlying angina to return, or it may precipitate a MI.

CRITICAL THINKING AND APPLICATION

Answer the following questions on a separate sheet of paper.

6. Mrs. Wong, a patient on your hospital floor, is receiving dopamine IV. When you first come on the late-night shift, she seems just fine. However, the next time you check on her you notice that the drug has leaked out. What could happen as a result? Is this serious? What kind of treatment do you recommend? Describe the unusual injection process and its rationale.

7. Mr. Cortis has had a myocardial infarction. He is told that he will be prescribed a "cardioprotective agent." He asks you to explain. Why can some beta-blockers be said to "protect" the heart?

8. Ms. Clarkson has been prescribed a beta-blocker. She is about to be released from the hospital, but first, her nurse gives her instructions about taking her apical pulse for 1 full minute, as well as her blood pressure. Why? What should she be looking for? Is there anything she should be instructed to report to her physician?

Copyright © 2002 by Mosby, Inc. All rights reserved.

Chapter 18

Cholinergic Agents

Match each definition with its corresponding term. (Note: Not all terms will be used.)

1. _____ Antidote for overdose of a cholinergic agent.

2. _____ Cholinergic drugs that act by making more ACh available at the receptor site, thus allowing ACh to bind to and stimulate the receptor.

3. _____ Cholinergic drugs that bind to cholinergic receptors and activate them.

4. _____ Receptors located postsynaptically in smooth muscle, cardiac muscle, the glands of the parasympathetic fibers, and in the effector organs of the cholinergic sympathetic fibers.

5. _____ Receptors located in the ganglia of the PSNS and the SNS.

6. _____ A description of the action of the PSNS.

7. _____ The neurotransmitter responsible for the transmission of nerve impulses to the effector cells in the PSNS.

8. _____ The enzyme responsible for breaking down ACh.

a. cholinesterase

b. Muscarinic

c. catecholamine

d. "Fight or flight"

e. "Rest and digest"

f. Direct-acting cholinergic agents

g. Indirect-acting cholinergic agents

h. atropine

i. acetylcholine

j. Nicotinic

Choose the *best* answer for each of the following.

9. The desired effects of cholinergic drugs come from stimulation of which receptors?
   a. Muscarinic
   b. Nicotinic
   c. Cholinergic
   d. Ganglionic

10. Bethanechol, the only direct-acting cholinergic drug that can be taken orally, is used for:
    a. urinary incontinence.
    b. urinary retention.
    c. diarrhea.
    d. bladder spasms.

11. Which agent is used for the symptomatic treatment of myasthenia gravis?
    a. bethanechol
    b. tacrine
    c. donepezil
    d. physostigmine

Copyright © 2002 by Mosby, Inc. All rights reserved.

12. Mary's mother, Annie, who is 62, has started taking donepezil for early stages of Alzheimer's disease. Mary expresses relief that "there is finally a pill to cure Alzheimer's disease." What should guide your response?
    a. She should expect reversal of symptoms within a few days.
    b. Mary should increase the dosage if no improvement is noted.
    c. This drug is for symptomatic improvement but they should not expect a cure.
    d. If they had started the medication any later, no improvement would have been noted.

13. Early signs of a cholinergic crisis in a patient who may have inadvertently received an overdose would include all the following *except*:
    a. salivation.
    b. dry mouth.
    c. flushing of the skin.
    d. abdominal cramps.

CRITICAL THINKING AND APPLICATION

Answer the following questions on a separate sheet of paper.

14. Explain the effects of cholinergic poisoning by using the acronym SLUDGE.

15. Mrs. Sibanda has recently given birth to an 8-pound baby girl. Mrs. Sibanda seems healthy and comfortable, with few postpartum contractions or cramping. However, her abdomen is distended, and she has not been able to void her urine in the expected time.

    a. What drug is likely to be the drug of choice?

    b. Mrs. Sibanda is still unable to void her urine. Her urinary retention worsens and becomes painful, and when her physician is contacted, he recommends radiography to determine the presence of a stone in her urinary tract; his suspicions are confirmed. How much can the physician increase her dosage?

16. Mr. Keegan has been determined to have a high potential for a negative reaction to the cholinergic prescribed to him. However, his physician believes that the potential benefits are worth the risk.

    a. What reaction should you be closely monitoring Mr. Keegan for?

    b. In addition to close monitoring, what else can you do to be prepared?

17. Ms. Bethke has recently been diagnosed with myasthenia gravis and is taking medication for the treatment of symptoms associated with the disease. She asks you, "How much success can I expect?"

    a. What will you say?

    b. Tell her what kind of negative effects she should report to a physician.

Copyright © 2002 by Mosby, Inc. All rights reserved.

Chapter 19

Cholinergic-Blocking Agents

Choose the *best* answer for each of the following.

1. Before giving an anticholinergic agent, the nurse should check the patient's history for:
   a. glaucoma.
   b. mental disorders.
   c. gallbladder disease.
   d. diabetes mellitus.

2. Which drug is commonly used preoperatively to dry secretions and prevent vagal stimulation?
   a. atenolol
   b. atropine
   c. physostigmine
   d. scopolamine

3. Side effects to expect from anticholinergic agents include all of the following *except*:
   a. dilated pupils.
   b. urinary retention.
   c. dry mouth.
   d. diarrhea.

4. Elderly patients taking anticholinergics should be reminded that they are at risk for:
   a. hypothermia.
   b. fluid overload.
   c. heat stroke.
   d. angina.

5. Mellie is taking a cruise and has asked for a prescription for motion sickness. The physician orders Transderm-Scōp (scopolamine) patches. What is important to tell Mellie when teaching her about this drug?
   a. It can be applied anywhere on the upper body.
   b. It should be applied 4 to 5 hours before travel.
   c. It should be applied just before the cruise begins.
   d. The patch needs to be changed daily.

CRITICAL THINKING AND APPLICATION

Answer the following questions on a separate sheet of paper.

6. Carrie, age 63, is taking tolterodine (Detrol) for urinary urge incontinence. What would you tell her about the purpose of the drug? Are there any other patient teaching concerns?

7. Mrs. Olafson has been taking Robinul for treatment of her peptic ulcer. She comes in to see her physician and says, "My ulcer pains are just as bad, and they wake me up at night." What might be suggested for her?

8. Mr. Miller is brought into the emergency room conscious but with an overdose of a cholinergic blocker.

   a. Describe Mr. Miller's treatment.

   b. How will treatment be altered if Mr. Miller suddenly loses consciousness or suffers from the onset of convulsions?

   c. Finally, how should you respond if Mr. Miller begins having hallucinations related to the overdose?

Copyright © 2002 by Mosby, Inc. All rights reserved.

9. Mr. Hansen is taking dicyclomine (Bentyl) for irritable bowel syndrome. He calls the clinic and tells you that he would like to get his doctor's permission to take an antihistamine for his cold. What drug interactions might he expect?

Chapter 20

Positive Inotropic Agents

Choose the *best* answer for each of the following.

1. When monitoring patients who are taking digoxin, the serum level should be:
   a. 0.1 to 0.5 ng/ml.
   b. 0.5 to 2.0 ng/ml.
   c. 2.0 to 5.0 ng/ml.
   d. 5.0 to 8.4 ng/ml.

2. An antidote for digitalis toxicity is:
   a. vitamin K.
   b. atropine.
   c. Digibind.
   d. digitoxin.

3. Before giving oral digoxin, you find that the patient's apical pulse is 55. You should:
   a. give the dose.
   b. hold the dose.
   c. hold the dose and notify the physician.
   d. check the radial pulse.

4. During digoxin therapy, it is essential to monitor serum potassium levels because:
   a. low potassium levels increase the chance of digoxin toxicity.
   b. high potassium levels increase the chance of digoxin toxicity.
   c. low potassium levels cause an increase in heart rate.
   d. digoxin promotes the excretion of potassium in the kidneys.

5. When infusing amrinone, it is important to remember that:
   a. the medication should be mixed in saline before administration.
   b. the true color of IV amrinone is clear yellow.
   c. it is used for the patient with acute myocardial infarction.
   d. hypertension is the primary effect seen with excessive doses.

CRITICAL THINKING AND APPLICATION

Answer the following questions on a separate sheet of paper.

6. You are caring for Mrs. Chin, who is undergoing cardiac glycoside therapy. She begins to vomit and complains of a headache and fatigue. Studies reveal a dysrhythmia and a serum potassium level of 6 mEq/L. What action might you expect to be taken?

7. Mr. Davis has atrial fibrillation and flutter, and the physician initially prescribes digoxin IV at 1.5 mg/day. What is the purpose of this dose, and how does it compare with the dose on which Mr. Davis will be maintained?

8. How does the concept of a therapeutic window relate to the monitoring of patients taking cardiac glycosides?

9. While monitoring Mr. Ferris following oral digoxin administration, you note the following: increased urinary output, decreased dyspnea and fatigue, and constipation. Mr. Ferris complains to you that if he were allowed to eat bran as often as he used to, he wouldn't be constipated. What do your findings indicate? What is your response to Mr. Ferris?

Copyright © 2002 by Mosby, Inc. All rights reserved.

10. Mr. Montgomery is experiencing heart failure that has not responded well to diuretic and digoxin therapy. The physician changes his medication to amrinone.

   a. What effect does amrinone have on cardiac muscle contractility and the blood vessels?

   b. What advantage does this phosphodiesterase inhibitor have over the cardiac glycosides?

   c. What is the most worrisome side effect of amrinone?

Copyright © 2002 by Mosby, Inc. All rights reserved.

Chapter 21

Antidysrhythmic Agents

Choose the *best* answer for each of the following.

1. The antidysrhythmic drug lidocaine is used mainly for the treatment of:
   a. atrial fibrillation.
   b. bradycardia.
   c. complete heart block.
   d. ventricular dysrhythmias.

2. When monitoring the patient who is taking quinidine, which finding would be a possible adverse effect of this drug?
   a. Hypokalemia
   b. Tachycardia
   c. Prolonged QT interval
   d. Hypertension

3. Possible adverse effects of amiodarone include all the following *except*:
   a. pulmonary toxicity.
   b. hypothyroidism.
   c. urinary retention.
   d. visual halos.

4. Verapamil is used mainly for:
   a. ventricular dysrhythmias, including PVCs.
   b. cardiac asystole.
   c. preventing and converting recurrent PSVT.
   d. heart blocks.

5. When giving adenosine, it is important to remember to:
   a. give it as a fast IV push.
   b. give it IV push slowly, over 5 minutes.
   c. offer it with food or milk.
   d. prepare to set up for an IV drip infusion.

CRITICAL THINKING AND APPLICATION

Answer the following questions on a separate sheet of paper.

6. Mr. Killian, who has been diagnosed with hypertension, is hospitalized following an MI.

   a. To reduce the risk of sudden cardiac death in Mr. Killian, the physician prescribes a drug from which class? Why?

   b. How would a history of asthma in Mr. Killian affect the drug choice?

   c. What if he had myasthenia gravis?

7. Mr. Needham has a life-threatening ventricular tachycardia that has been resistant to treatment, and the physician has now prescribed what she calls a "last resort" drug. What drug is she referring to, and why is it considered a drug of last resort?

8. Ms. Lionel, a 56-year-old homemaker, is being treated for PSVT, and the physician prescribes verapamil.

   a. Ms. Lionel is very concerned about her treatment and asks you, "Why did my doctor take away my high blood pressure medication?" What is your answer?

69

Copyright © 2002 by Mosby, Inc. All rights reserved.

b. Ms. Lionel is not responding to the verapamil as the physician had hoped. What action might the nurse expect to be taken next?

9. Mr. Maxwell is a 50-year-old schoolteacher being treated with lidocaine following an MI. He is very agitated and says that he hates injections; he wants to know why he can't just take a pill. He also asks you for more blankets because he feels shaky and cold. What action do you take?

10. Mrs. Inez calls the health clinic complaining of chest pain and dizziness. She says she can't remember whether she took her quinidine yesterday and wants to know whether she should take two doses today, especially because she is feeling so bad. What do you tell Mrs. Inez?

Copyright © 2002 by Mosby, Inc. All rights reserved.

Chapter 22

Antianginal Agents

Choose the *best* answer for each of the following.

1. The purpose of antianginal drug therapy is to:
   a. increase myocardial oxygen demand.
   b. decrease myocardial oxygen demand.
   c. increase blood flow to ischemic myocardium.
   d. decrease blood flow to ischemic myocardium.

2. Which is a common side effect of nitroglycerin?
   a. Blurred vision
   b. Dizziness
   c. Headache
   d. Weakness

3. Nitroglycerin is available in all the following forms *except*:
   a. transdermal patch.
   b. IV bolus.
   c. sublingual spray.
   d. topical ointment.

4. What is the best way to prevent tolerance to nitrates when using the transdermal patches?
   a. Leave the old patch on for 2 hours when applying a new patch.
   b. Apply a new patch every other day.
   c. Leave the patch off for 24 hours once a week.
   d. Remove the patch at night for 8 hours then apply a new patch in the morning.

5. Patients who are taking beta-blockers for angina need to be taught that:
   a. these drugs are for long-term prevention of angina, not immediate relief of pain.
   b. they should be taken as soon as pain is present.
   c. they should discontinue the medication if they experience dizziness or tiredness.
   d. measures to prevent diarrhea need to be taken.

CRITICAL THINKING AND APPLICATION

Answer the following questions on a separate sheet of paper.

6. You are playing racquetball at a community center when you notice a commotion at a gathering of senior citizens in a nearby room. You rush in to find a man lying unconscious on the floor. Several people say that he is having a "heart attack." One man hands you a vial and asks, "Would it help to give him one of my heart pills?" A woman agrees, saying, "Yes! Can't you put it under his tongue?" Someone else offers a second vial, encouraging you to put one of those pills under the victim's tongue. You see that the first vial is labeled Peritrate, the second Isordil. What do you know about these medications, and what should you do?

7. Ms. Vickers is a 70-year-old woman seen in the ER for a laceration to her thumb. During your assessment, Ms. Vickers tells you that she's been "tired and depressed" and has been having "nightmares" since her doctor prescribed heart medicine for her angina. Which drug do you suspect Ms. Vickers is taking? Why do you think so?

8. During your home visit with Theresa, she shows you a journal entry describing the duration, time of onset, and severity of a recent angina attack. She reports no adverse effects to her nitroglycerin and shows you where she keeps the tablets: in a clear plastic pillbox on the kitchen windowsill. What do you discuss with Theresa?

71

Copyright © 2002 by Mosby, Inc. All rights reserved.

Chapter 23

Antihypertensive Agents

CRITICAL THINKING CROSSWORD

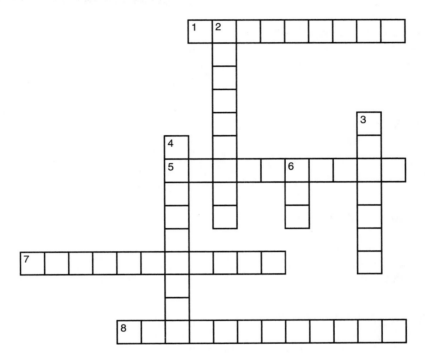

Across

1. High blood pressure associated with several primary diseases, such as renal, pulmonary, endocrine, and vascular diseases, is known as _____ hypertension.
5. Another term for 3 Down.
7. Common side effect of adrenergic drugs involving a sudden drop in blood pressure when patients change position is known as _____ hypotension.
8. Used in the management of hypertensive emergencies.

Down

2. Another term for 3 Down.
3. Elevated systemic arterial pressure for which no cause can be found is known as _____ hypertension.
4. The primary effect of these agents is to decrease plasma and extracellular fluid volumes.
6. Agents that are often used as first-line agents in the treatment of both CHF and hypertension are known as angiotensin-converting enzyme inhibitors, or _____ inhibitors.

Copyright © 2002 by Mosby, Inc. All rights reserved.

Choose the *best* answer for each of the following.

1. Michael, age 46, has been taking clonidine for 5 months, and his blood pressure has been normal for the last 2 months. He tells you that he would like to stop taking the drug. What should you say?
   a. "Go ahead and stop it—your blood pressure is normal now."
   b. "Stop taking the drug for a month, and we'll see how you do."
   c. "This drug should not be stopped suddenly; let's talk to your doctor."
   d. "You can stop the drug if you exercise and avoid salty foods."

2. All of the following side effects may occur with the use of ACE inhibitors *except*:
   a. a dry, nonproductive cough.
   b. fatigue.
   c. restlessness.
   d. headaches.

3. Reserpine is often prescribed with diuretics because:
   a. diuretics enhance the action of reserpine.
   b. the antihypertensive effect of reserpine may diminish with continued use.

   c. a lower dose of reserpine may then be given.
   d. diuretics may counteract the side effects that often occur with reserpine.

4. Which drug would be used for a hypertensive emergency?
   a. sodium nitroprusside
   b. losartan
   c. captopril
   d. prazosin

5. Julie, who is in the 8th month of pregnancy, has preeclampsia, and her blood pressure is 210/100 this morning. She has which type of hypertension?
   a. Primary
   b. Idiopathic
   c. Essential
   d. Secondary

CRITICAL THINKING AND APPLICATION

Answer the following questions on a separate sheet of paper.

6. Mr. Quester, 61 years of age, came in to the emergency room last night with symptoms of severe hypertensive emergency. The ER resident on call put him on trimethaphan camsylate. This morning, when Mr. Quester's regular physician paid his first visit, he switched him to "one of the newer drugs." Why?

7. In an emergency, Ms. Peck is put on trimethaphan to lower her blood pressure.
   a. Describe the administration procedure.
   b. You learn that she is to be taken off the medication within 24 hours; a switch is planned. Why?

8. Identify which ACE inhibitor would be best for the following patients. Explain your answers.
   a. Irene, who has liver dysfunction, as well as high blood pressure, and who is seriously ill.
   b. Kory, who has a history of poor compliance with his medication regimen.

9. Mr. Bass will be starting prazosin for hypertension. What should he be taught before he takes even the first dose of this medication?

Copyright © 2002 by Mosby, Inc. All rights reserved.

Chapter 24

Diuretic Agents

Match each term with its corresponding definition.

1. _____ Diuretics

2. _____ Potassium-sparing diuretics

3. _____ Kaliuretic diuretics

4. _____ Osmotic diuretics

5. _____ Thiazides

6. _____ Ascites

7. _____ CAIs

8. _____ Loop diuretics

a. Potent diuretics that act along the ascending limb of the loop of Henle; furosemide is an example.

b. A class of diuretics that inhibits the enzyme carbonic anhydrase; acetazolamide is an example.

c. A general term for drugs that accelerate the rate of urine formation.

d. A term for diuretics that cause the body to lose potassium.

e. Diuretics that result in the diuresis of sodium and water and the retention of potassium; spironolactone is an example.

f. Diuretics that act on the distal convoluted tubule where they inhibit sodium and water resorption; HCTZ is an example.

g. Agents that induce diuresis by increasing the osmotic pressure of the glomerular filtrate, resulting in a rapid diuresis; mannitol is an example.

h. An abnormal intraperitoneal accumulation of fluid.

Choose the *best* answer for each of the following.

9. All of the following are indications for the use of diuretics *except*:
   a. increased urine output.
   b. reduced uric acid levels.
   c. treatment of hypertension.
   d. treatment of edema associated with heart failure.

10. Marvin is taking spironolactone (Aldactone). What dietary guidelines should he follow?
    a. There are no dietary restrictions with this medication.
    b. He should eat foods high in potassium, such as bananas and orange juice.
    c. He should avoid foods high in potassium.
    d. He should drink 1 to 2 liters of fluid per day.

11. When teaching the patient about diuretic therapy, what is the optimal time of day for administration of these medications?
    a. Morning
    b. Mid-day
    c. Bedtime
    d. Time of day does not matter

12. Which of the following may indicate hypokalemia, a possible side effect of diuretics?
    a. Nausea, vomiting, anorexia
    b. Diarrhea and abdominal pain
    c. Orthostatic hypotension
    d. Muscle weakness and lethargy

Copyright © 2002 by Mosby, Inc. All rights reserved.

13. Which of the following groups of diuretics are
    not recommended to reduce edema?
    a. Loop diuretics
    b. CAI
    c. Osmotic diuretics
    d. Thiazides

CRITICAL THINKING AND APPLICATION

Answer the following questions on a separate sheet of paper.

14. Ms. Andersen is a 62-year-old retired teacher who is being treated for diabetes and open-angle glaucoma. The physician has prescribed a diuretic as an adjunct agent in the management of Ms. Andersen's glaucoma.

    a. Which diuretic agent was probably prescribed?

    b. What undesirable effect of the agent does the physician need to consider?

15. You are about to administer mannitol to Arthur, who is in early acute renal failure.

    a. What is the significance of Arthur's renal blood flow and glomerular filtration in this situation?

    b. By what means do you administer the mannitol? What special guidelines do you follow?

    c. Arthur later complains of a headache and chills. Should the mannitol therapy be terminated? Explain your answer.

16. Mr. Ferrara has been admitted to your unit for treatment of ascites. He also has some renal impairment and a history of heavy drinking.

    a. Which diuretic agent do you expect to be administered to Mr. Ferrara?

    b. What monitoring will be performed frequently? Why?

17. Brendan, a 39-year-old bricklayer, is taking thiazide for hypertension. During a follow-up visit, he tells you that he thinks the drug is affecting his "love life."

    a. What side effect of thiazide therapy is Brendan probably referring to?

    b. While you're talking, you notice a package of licorice in Brendan's coat pocket. He tells you he eats the candy "for energy," especially because he has been feeling so tired the past couple of days. What do you tell Brendan?

18. You receive a call from Mrs. Hill, who was recently started on diuretic therapy for hypertension. Mrs. Hill is concerned because her neighbor, who also takes medication for hypertension, has told her not to eat a lot of bananas or other foods containing potassium. "But you told me to eat foods high in potassium," Mrs. Hill says to you. "What's going on?" What is your response to Mrs. Hill?

19. a. Why should patients undergoing diuretic therapy monitor their daily weight?

    b. What change in weight should be reported to the physician immediately?

    c. Why should vomiting and/or diarrhea be reported to the physician?

Copyright © 2002 by Mosby, Inc. All rights reserved.

Chapter 25

Fluids and Electrolytes

Choose the *best* answer for each of the following.

1. Common uses for crystalloids include all the following *except*:
   a. to replace fluids when there are body fluid deficits.
   b. to promote urinary flow.
   c. as maintenance fluids.
   d. to carry oxygen in the fluid.

2. Which concentration of sodium chloride is considered hypertonic?
   a. 0.33%
   b. 0.45%
   c. 0.9%
   d. 3.0%

3. In what way are colloids superior to crystalloids?
   a. Colloids have a better ability to expand the peripheral volume.
   b. Crystalloids are more likely to promote bleeding.
   c. Colloids do not contain protein, which prevent water from leaving the plasma.
   d. Colloids supply sodium and water to maintain fluid volume.

4. When giving IV potassium, it is important to remember that:
   a. IV doses are preferred over oral dosage forms.
   b. IV solutions should contain at least 50 mEq/L.
   c. it must always be given in diluted form.
   d. it should be given by slow IV bolus.

5. When a patient is receiving blood products, what are the signs of a possible transfusion reaction?
   a. Subnormal temperature and hypertension
   b. Apprehension, restlessness, fever, and chills
   c. Decreased pulse and respirations and fever
   d. Headache, nausea, and lethargy

CRITICAL THINKING AND APPLICATION

Answer the following questions on a separate sheet of paper.

6. How does albumin differ from the other colloids in terms of its particle composition and metabolization?

7. a. Which fluids are also called oxygen-carrying resuscitation fluids?

   b. Why are these fluids able to carry oxygen?

   c. Why are they the most expensive of the three types of fluids, and why is their origin a potential problem for a recipient?

Copyright © 2002 by Mosby, Inc. All rights reserved.

8. Tanya, a 16-year-old student, is brought to the clinic by her mother, who says that Tanya has been on "some sort of fad diet." The mother is concerned because Tanya is tired and weak. During your assessment, Tanya admits that she has been using laxatives and eating very little the past few weeks.

   a.   What electrolyte imbalance is Tanya probably experiencing?

   b.   Assuming that laboratory studies show the problem to be mild, how can it be corrected?

9. Mr. Sanchez, a 45-year-old mail carrier, has come to the ER sweating profusely and complaining of stomach cramps and diarrhea. He says that he has been "miserable" from the heat the past few days. His serum sodium level is 131 mEq/L.

   a.   What electrolyte imbalance do you suspect?

   b.   The physician prescribes an oral medication and then asks you to discuss dietary considerations with Mr. Sanchez. What do you tell Mr. Sanchez?

   c.   What symptom is Mr. Sanchez now experiencing that is also a side effect of the medication he has been prescribed?

10. Victor is receiving a transfusion of a blood product.

   a.   You observe Victor, knowing that a source of early evidence of an adverse reaction to the transfusion is what?

   b.   Victor's wife is crying and says, "People get AIDS from transfusions. What happens if Victor gets AIDS?" What do you tell her?

   c.   The transfusion for Victor seems to be progressing smoothly. How often do you check Victor's vital signs while he is receiving the transfusion?

   d.   After 45 minutes, Victor is restless, and his pulse has increased. What do you do?

Copyright © 2002 by Mosby, Inc. All rights reserved.

Chapter 26

Coagulation Modifier Agents

Match each definition with its corresponding term. (Note: Not all terms will be used.)

1. _____ A drug that prevents the lysis of fibrin, thereby promoting clot formation.

2. _____ The termination of bleeding by mechanical or chemical means.

3. _____ A substance that prevents platelet plugs from forming.

4. _____ A drug or other agent that dissolves thrombi.

5. _____ A substance that prevents or delays coagulation of the blood.

6. _____ A laboratory test used to measure the effectiveness of heparin therapy.

7. _____ A laboratory test used to measure the effectiveness of warfarin sodium therapy.

8. _____ This substance reverses the effect of heparin.

9. _____ This substance reverses the effect of warfarin sodium.

10. _____ Naturally occurring t-PA secreted by vascular endothelial cells.

11. _____ A blood clot that dislodges and travels through the bloodstream.

a. Prothrombin time

b. APTT

c. Streptokinase

d. alteplase (Activase)

e. Thrombus

f. Embolus

g. Vitamin K

h. protamine sulfate

i. Antiplatelet drug

j. Antifibrinolytic

k. Thrombolytic agent

l. Anticoagulant

m. Hemostasis

Choose the *best* answer for each of the following.

12. Which of the following conditions would *not* be appropriate for the use of anticoagulants?
    a. Atrial fibrillation
    b. Aneurysms
    c. Myocardial infarction
    d. Presence of mechanical heart valves

13. When teaching the patient who will be taking warfarin sodium (Coumadin) at home, what should the patient be told regarding OTC drug use?
    a. Choose NSAIDs over aspirin as needed for pain relief.
    b. Aspirin and other NSAIDs may result in increased anticoagulant effect.

c. Vitamin E therapy is recommended to improve the effect of the Coumadin.
d. Mineral oil is the laxative of choice while taking anticoagulants.

14. Which agent has antiplatelet properties?
    a. aspirin
    b. enoxaparin
    c. heparin
    d. urokinase

Copyright © 2002 by Mosby, Inc. All rights reserved.

15. When administering subcutaneous heparin, the nurse should remember to:
    a. use the same sites for injection to reduce trauma.
    b. use a 1-inch needle for subcutaneous injections.
    c. remove the needle after the injection, without aspirating.
    d. rub the site after the injection to increase absorption.

16. Which symptoms may indicate a serious bleeding problem during thrombolytic therapy and should be reported to the physician immediately?
    a. Decreased blood pressure and restlessness
    b. Increased blood pressure and decreased pulse rate
    c. Increased lethargy and dizziness
    d. Epistaxis and decreased pulse rate

CRITICAL THINKING AND APPLICATION

Answer the following questions on a separate sheet of paper.

17. Mrs. Washington, a 60-year-old homemaker, is undergoing heparin therapy for deep vein thrombosis.

    a. After you give Mrs. Washington her injection, she complains of pain and begins to rub the site. Is that a problem?

    b. What is the most commonly used test for determining the effects of heparin therapy?

18. During cardiopulmonary bypass for heart surgery, Mr. Wong was intentionally given a large dose of heparin. The surgeon then determines that the effects of the heparin need to be reversed quickly.

    a. How will this be done?

    b. How will the amount of antidote be determined?

19. If vitamin K is warfarin sodium's reversal agent, how can its use cause a problem for a patient experiencing warfarin toxicity?

20. Following surgery, Mr. Thurman has a chest tube in place. The site has been bleeding excessively.

    a. What type of agent might the physician prescribe in this situation and why?

    b. How, and in what dosage, do you expect to administer the drug?

21. William, a 38-year-old writer who has von Willebrand's disease, has undergone emergency surgery following an automobile accident. What agent is used in the management of bleeding in patients like William? What is its effect?

22. Tobias has been given Activase during his treatment for AMI.

    a. Do you expect Tobias to have an allergic reaction to the agent? Explain your answer.

    b. A few minutes later, Tobias suffers a reinfarction. What agent should Tobias receive now?

23. Ursula, an inpatient on your unit, is on anticoagulant therapy. You enter her room to find that she is restless and confused.

    a. Why are these findings significant?

    b. In this case, what other problems might you expect to find?

    c. What should you do?

Copyright © 2002 by Mosby, Inc. All rights reserved.

Chapter 27

Antilipemic Agents

Choose the *best* answer for each of the following.

1. Patients taking cholestyramine may experience which of the following side effects?
   a. Blurred vision and photophobia
   b. Drowsiness and difficulty concentrating
   c. Diarrhea and abdominal cramps
   d. Belching and bloating

2. Dietary concerns for the patient on antilipemic therapy include all the following *except*:
   a. supplemental fat-soluble vitamins.
   b. supplemental B-vitamin complex, especially niacin.
   c. increasing the intake of high-fiber foods.
   d. choosing and preparing foods that are lower in cholesterol and saturated fats.

3. The presence of which condition is a contraindication to the use of antilipemic therapy?
   a. Liver disease
   b. Renal disease
   c. Coronary artery disease
   d. Diabetes mellitus

4. A concern with probucol therapy is that:
   a. it decreases LDL levels.
   b. it decreases HDL levels.
   c. it is not generally well-tolerated.
   d. it is very expensive.

5. Undesirable side effects of niacin may be minimized by:
   a. starting niacin at full-strength to help the patient build tolerance.
   b. taking niacin on an empty stomach.
   c. taking a small dose of NSAIDs 30 minutes before the niacin.
   d. taking the niacin every other day if side effects are bothersome.

6. For each of the following drugs, name the antilipemic category and briefly describe how the drug lowers lipid levels.

   a. fenofibrate (Tricor)

   b. niacin

   c. lovastatin (Mevacor)

   d. cholestyramine (Questran)

CRITICAL THINKING AND APPLICATION

Answer the following questions on a separate sheet of paper.

7. Mr. Harris is a 46-year-old business executive who travels frequently. He is slightly overweight "from all that room service," but he did quit smoking 6 years ago. During a routine checkup, Mr. Harris is found to have an LDL cholesterol level of 230. He says, "I'm a busy man! Just give me some pills. I've got a plane to catch!" Will the physician prescribe an antilipemic for Mr. Harris? Explain your answer.

81

Copyright © 2002 by Mosby, Inc. All rights reserved.

8. Mr. Jahnke is a 49-year-old farmer. During assessment, you discover the following: Mr. Jahnke's mother is living, but his father "dropped dead of a heart attack" at the age of 53. Mr. Jahnke is a smoker with mild asthma and some arthritis in his hands. His blood pressure today is 138/78, and laboratory studies show an HDL of 67 mg/dl. Discuss Mr. Jahnke's risk factors for high cholesterol.

9. Mrs. Kim has been treated with cholestyramine for type IIa hyperlipidemia for the past 2 months. She tells you that she "can't stand being so irregular" and that she has developed another "embarrassing problem" as well. What is wrong with Mrs. Kim, and how can you help her?

10. Justus is a 55-year-old attorney being treated with lovastatin for his hyperlipidemia. His current health history includes mild hypertension and a peptic ulcer. You know that niacin is frequently prescribed as an adjunct to other antilipemic agents. Would niacin be helpful for Justus? Explain your answer.

11. You are visiting Mrs. Nguyen, a homebound patient who is being treated for hyperlipidemia and hypertension. During your visit, Mrs. Nguyen takes her antihypertensive and then begins stirring her dose of Questran into a glass of orange juice. What patient teaching does Mrs. Nguyen require?

Copyright © 2002 by Mosby, Inc. All rights reserved.

Chapter 28

Pituitary Agents

1. Complete the following table.

Hormone	Function	Mimicking Drug(s)
Adrenocorticotropic hormone	Targets adrenal gland; mediates adaptation to stressors; promotes synthesis of these three hormones: **a.**	**b.**
Growth hormone	**c.**	**d.**
e.	Increases water resorption in distal tubules and collecting duct of nephron; concentrates urine.	**f.**

Choose the *best* answer for each of the following.

2. Uses for corticotropin include all the following *except*:
   a. diagnosis of adrenocortical insufficiency.
   b. treatment of multiple sclerosis.
   c. stimulating skeletal growth.
   d. as an antiinflammatory agent.

3. Which agent is used in the treatment of type I von Willebrand's disease or hemophilia A?
   a. corticotropin
   b. vasopressin
   c. octreotide
   d. desmopressin

4. Which nursing diagnosis may be appropriate for the patient who is receiving a pituitary agent?
   a. Deficient fluid volume
   b. Disturbed body image
   c. Impaired physical mobility
   d. Impaired skin integrity

5. When receiving desmopressin acetate as a nasal spray for diabetes insipidus, which action would provide optimal control of the patient's disease?
   a. Clear the nasal passages after spraying the medication.
   b. Inhale the spray for full drug effect.
   c. If nasal congestion occurs, take an OTC preparation to control mucus.
   d. Take the nasal spray at the same time every day.

6. Which hormone is secreted by the posterior pituitary gland?
   a. antidiuretic hormone (ADH)
   b. aldosterone
   c. growth hormone
   d. thyroid-stimulating hormone

83

Copyright © 2002 by Mosby, Inc. All rights reserved.

CRITICAL THINKING AND APPLICATION

Answer the following questions on a separate sheet of paper.

7. Alexis has multiple sclerosis. She is experiencing pain associated with inflammation.

   a. What drug might the physician recommend for Alexis? What else might this drug provide besides pain relief?

   b. What cautions—and/or contraindications—should you look for before this drug is administered?

   c. What else might you include in assessing Alexis for treatment?

   d. Alexis is determined to be an appropriate candidate for this drug of choice. Draw up an appropriate patient teaching plan.

8. You have recently begun working in a specialized endocrinology clinic. Your first patient, Patricia, a second grader, is not growing at the rate that is expected. The physician has determined that Patricia is a candidate for somatropin. Her parents are nervous about giving injections to Patricia. What should be emphasized while teaching her parents about giving this drug?

9. Mr. Collins has been experiencing severe thirst, which, "of course, makes me go to the bathroom all the time, it seems like."

   a. Predict Mr. Collins' likely disorder and two likely drugs of choice for Mr. Collins.

   b. How will you assess Mr. Collins before administering these drugs?

   c. As a result of your thorough assessment, it has been determined that Mr. Collins should do well with lypressin therapy. Describe the treatment and its therapeutic effects (that is, how it mimics the natural hormone) to the patient.

   d. Following your explanation Mr. Collins says, "Okay, okay, but what does it do for me?" Explain the physical improvements Mr. Collins should be able to see.

   e. Mr. Collins begins therapy. Draw up a teaching plan for him. Take this opportunity to warn him about side effects and adverse reactions for which he should be on the lookout.

Copyright © 2002 by Mosby, Inc. All rights reserved.

Chapter 29

Thyroid and Antithyroid Agents

CRITICAL THINKING CROSSWORD

Across

3. The type of hypothyroidism that results from insufficient secretion of TSH from the pituitary gland.
6. Thyroid hormone that influences the metabolic rate.
7. The type of hypothyroidism that is due to the inability of the thyroid gland to perform a function.

Down

1. The most commonly prescribed synthetic thyroid hormone.
2. Excessive secretion of thyroid hormones.
4. An agent used to treat hyperthyroidism.
5. The type of hypothyroidism that stems from reduced levels of TRH secreted from the hypothalamus.
6. Another name for TSH.

Copyright © 2002 by Mosby, Inc. All rights reserved.

Choose the *best* answer for each of the following.

1. Patients who begin therapy with levothyroxine should be told to expect effects from the medication:
   a. immediately.
   b. within a few days.
   c. within a few weeks.
   d. within a few months.

2. Mrs. Smith wants to switch brands of levothyroxine. What is your response?
   a. Different brands are metabolized at different rates.
   b. Each brand has a different ratio of T_3 and T_4.
   c. There should be no difference in the therapeutic response among different brands.
   d. She should consult her physician before switching brands.

3. The patient on antithyroid medications should be advised to avoid which foods?
   a. Soy products and seafood
   b. Bananas and oranges
   c. Dairy products
   d. Processed meats and cheese

4. When teaching patients about taking thyroid medications, which of the following is *not* true?
   a. A log or journal of their responses, and a graph of their pulse, weight, and mood would be helpful.
   b. They should discontinue the medication if side effects become too strong.
   c. The medication should be taken at the same time every day.
   d. Nervousness, irritability, and insomnia may be a result of a dose that is too high.

5. Mr. T. is scheduled for a radioactive isotope study. He takes levothyroxine daily; what instructions regarding his medications should he receive from his health care provider?
   a. Continue to take the medication as ordered.
   b. Skip the medication on the morning of the test.
   c. Stop the medication about 4 weeks before the test.
   d. Reduce the dosage 1 week before the test.

CRITICAL THINKING AND APPLICATION

Answer the following questions on a separate sheet of paper.

6. Mrs. Westin, age 43, comes into the clinic complaining of hair loss, lethargy, and constipation. "I just can't eat anything," she says. As you take her blood pressure, you notice that her skin feels thickened. Which of the disorders discussed in this chapter is Mrs. Westin most likely to have? Suggest several possible appropriate medications. Which of those is generally preferred? Why?

7. Ms. Hilton has had Graves' disease for 3 years. Today she reports symptoms of diarrhea, muscle weakness, fatigue, and palpitations. Also, she says, despite the diarrhea, she often has an increased appetite. She is also having trouble sleeping and wonders whether she's undergoing menopause because she suffers flushing, heat intolerance, and altered menstrual flow. As you ask her questions about these symptoms, you note that she seems irritable. This is understandable given her multiple symptoms; however, you have known Ms. Hilton since she began treatment for Graves' disease, and she has always been far from irritable, no matter how she felt. What's going on here?

8. Your suspicions are confirmed by the physician. Ms. Hilton is started on methimazole PO 60 mg/day in 3 divided doses. Later, when the condition is under control, she is switched to a reduced maintenance dose of 10 mg/day. Finally, one day, after a couple of years have passed, Ms. Hilton returns for a routine follow-up and tells you she is delighted. "All of my symptoms have cleared up," she says, "and I'm cured!" What do you need to explain to Ms. Hilton about the therapeutic effects of methimazole, especially as it pertains to her case?

Copyright © 2002 by Mosby, Inc. All rights reserved.

Chapter 30

Antidiabetic and Hypoglycemic Agents

Choose the *best* answer for each of the following.

1. What is the most immediate and serious adverse effect of insulin therapy?
   a. Hyperglycemia
   b. Hypoglycemia
   c. Bradycardia
   d. Weakness

2. Which insulin has the longest duration?
   a. Regular
   b. Lente
   c. NPH
   d. Ultra Lente

3. Which type of insulin can be given intravenously?
   a. Regular
   b. Lente
   c. NPH
   d. Ultra Lente

4. Which of the following indicates hypoglycemia?
   a. Decreased pulse and respirations and flushed skin
   b. Increased pulse rate and a fruity, acetone breath odor
   c. Weakness, cold clammy skin, and shallow, rapid breathing
   d. Increased urine output and edema

5. When administering oral antidiabetic agents, which of the following is true?
   a. Administer them 30 minutes before meals.
   b. Administer them with meals.
   c. Administer them on an empty stomach.
   d. Administer them 1 hour after eating.

6. Which statement describes the mechanism of action of rosiglitazone (Avandia)?
   a. It stimulates beta cells to produce insulin.
   b. It decreases insulin resistance.
   c. It inhibits hepatic glucose production.
   d. It increases the sensitivity of peripheral tissue to insulin.

CRITICAL THINKING AND APPLICATION

Answer the following questions on a separate sheet of paper.

7. Describe the recommended rotation technique for insulin injections.

8. Alice has mild hypoglycemia. Her physician has recommended dietary modifications to treat the condition.

   a. What general dietary guidelines should she follow?

   b. You know that one of the early signs of hypoglycemia is irritability. Why is this true?

   c. What is the treatment for hypoglycemia?

Copyright © 2002 by Mosby, Inc. All rights reserved.

9. Your co-worker Bill is in the medications room preparing a dose of Novolin-R to administer to a patient on your unit.

   a. Before he administers the medication, how should Bill verify the order?

   b. When you enter the room, you notice that the insulin is cloudy. When you tell Bill to discard it, he says, "Insulin is supposed to look this way." Who is right, you or Bill?

   c. You examine the vial. A date on the label indicates that it has been on the shelf in this room for 2 months. Why is that a problem?

10. Alec is a 20-year-old student at a private Jewish university in a large city. He has been diagnosed with type 1 diabetes. The physician determines that Alec would be best treated with an insulin product that has an onset of 1 or 2 hours and a duration of 24 hours.

    a. What type of insulin does Alec require?

    b. What else might the physician need to consider when choosing a specific agent for Alec?

11. Mrs. Franklin, a 48-year-old homemaker, is 5 feet tall and weighs 180 pounds. During a routine physical, laboratory studies indicate an elevated blood glucose level. Your assessment of Mrs. Franklin reveals that she is a smoker with mild hypertension. The physician suspects type 2 diabetes.

    a. What initial treatment is indicated for Mrs. Franklin? Explain your answer.

    b. At a follow-up visit 3 months later, Mrs. Franklin's blood glucose level is still elevated. She has quit smoking, however, and has been walking for exercise. What treatment is indicated now?

12. Dennis is a 40-year-old cab company dispatcher who takes Diabinese. He comes to the ER late one Sunday evening complaining that he feels weak and that his face "feels hot." You note that Dennis has profound flushing, is sweating, and has an increased respiratory rate.

    a. What is Dennis exhibiting the signs and symptoms of?

    b. What may have caused it? How can you tell?

13. The physician is planning to prescribe a second-generation sulfonylurea agent for Mr. Dressel, a 50-year-old financial advisor with a history of frequent kidney infections. In particular, Mr. Dressel requires treatment for the short-term elevation in his blood glucose level that occurs after he eats.

    a. Why did the physician choose a second-generation sulfonylurea rather than, for example, chlorpropamide?

    b. Which second-generation sulfonylurea will the physician prescribe, and why?

    c. A few weeks later Mr. Dressel is vomiting and has been unable to eat for several hours. What should he do, and why?

Copyright © 2002 by Mosby, Inc. All rights reserved.

Chapter 31

Adrenal Agents

Choose the *best* answer for each of the following.

1. Jonathan has been taking prednisone following a severe reaction to poison ivy. He notices that the dosage of the medication decreases; he asks you why he must continue the medication and why he can't just stop taking it now that the skin rash is better. What is the best response?
   a. Sudden discontinuation of this medication may cause an adrenal crisis.
   b. He would experience withdrawal symptoms if the drug is discontinued abruptly.
   c. Cushing's syndrome may develop as a reaction to a sudden drop of serum cortisone levels.
   d. He can stop taking the medication if his rash is better.

2. Which medication is the preferred oral glucocorticoid for antiinflammatory or immunosuppressant purposes?
   a. Florinef
   b. dexamethasone
   c. prednisone
   d. hydrocortisone

3. Side effects of prednisone therapy include all the following *except*:
   a. fragile skin.
   b. increased glucose levels.
   c. nervousness.
   d. weight loss.

4. Which agent works to inhibit the function of the adrenal cortex in the treatment of Cushing's syndrome?
   a. dexamethasone
   b. aminoglutethimide
   c. hydrocortisone
   d. fludrocortisone

5. All of the following conditions are indications for the use of glucocorticoids except:
   a. organ transplant recipients.
   b. cerebral edema.
   c. bacterial infections.
   d. bronchospasm states.

CRITICAL THINKING AND APPLICATION

Answer the following questions on a separate sheet of paper.

6. Ms. Rivera, a 30-year-old hospital receptionist, is receiving glucocorticoid therapy following a kidney transplant. You are reviewing her drug regimen with her when she tells you that she frequently uses aspirin or Advil to treat problems like headaches or menstrual cramps. She also mentions that she enjoys walking for exercise and likes to visit sick children on the hospital's pediatric ward when she has time. What issues do you discuss with Ms. Rivera?

7. Peter, a 21-year-old mechanic, has developed a severe skin rash following a camping trip. The physician is planning to prescribe prednisone. Your nursing assessment reveals that Peter has diabetes.

   a. Does that finding affect Peter's treatment? Explain your answer.

   b. What advice, to help minimize GI effects, do you have for someone taking an oral form of the systemic adrenal agents?

Copyright © 2002 by Mosby, Inc. All rights reserved.

8. You are watching a student nurse prepare to apply a topical glucocorticoid to a patient's skin rash. After donning gloves, she places some of the medication on her finger. Should you intervene, or is the student nurse doing fine so far? What other consideration is involved in determining the technique for applying a topical agent?

9. Nina has been prescribed a steroid inhaler. What special instructions do you give her?

Copyright © 2002 by Mosby, Inc. All rights reserved.

Chapter 32

Women's Health Agents

Choose the *best* answer for each of the following.

1. All the following are contraindications to the use of oral contraceptives *except*:
   a. breast cancer.
   b. pregnancy.
   c. thrombophlebitic disorders.
   d. asthma.

2. Which of the following should be included when teaching about post-menopausal estrogen replacement therapy?
   a. Postmenopausal women are at a greater risk for gynecologic cancers.
   b. Oral forms should be taken on an empty stomach for best absorption.
   c. Taking an antacid with the estrogen may help with the GI upset.
   d. Supplemental calcium is not needed if the patient is taking estrogen.

3. When combination oral contraceptives are used to provide postcoital emergency contraception, which of the following statements is true?
   a. They are not effective if the woman is pregnant.
   b. They should be taken within 24 hours of unprotected intercourse.
   c. They are given in one dose.
   d. They are intended to terminate pregnancy.

4. Dinoprostone cervical gel is used to:
   a. induce abortion during the second trimester.
   b. improve cervical inducibility ("ripening") near term for labor induction.
   c. soften the cervix in women who are experiencing infertility problems.
   d. reduce postpartum uterine atony and hemorrhage.

5. Tocolytics such as terbutaline are used to prevent contractions:
   a. before the 20th week.
   b. between the 20th and 37th week.
   c. after the 37th week.
   d. at any time during the pregnancy if delivery is not desired.

CRITICAL THINKING AND APPLICATION

Answer the following questions on a separate sheet of paper.

6. Isabelle is a 48-year-old woman exhibiting symptoms of menopause. Assessment of Isabelle reveals a history of depression and mild arthritis.

   a. What do you need to ask Isabelle, and why?

   b. The physician decides to prescribe estrogen therapy. At this time, what do you know about the dose and the length of time it will be administered?

Copyright © 2002 by Mosby, Inc. All rights reserved.

7. Ms. Keller is a 25-year-old paralegal with diabetes. She is at the physician's office today because her menstrual periods have ceased. The physician has decided to prescribe a hormonal agent.

   a.   Which agent will the physician likely prescribe?

   b.   What adjustments to Ms. Keller's existing drug regimen might need to be made?

8. Jacklyn has been prescribed Ortho-Novum for birth control purposes. At a follow-up visit 4 months later, she tells you, "I am really messing up. I take the pills for 3 weeks, but when I'm off them for a week, sometimes I don't remember to start again!"

   a.   What might you suggest to help Jacklyn?

   b.   Jacklyn then expresses concern that her menstrual bleeding, now that she's on birth control pills, is "nothing compared with what it used to be." She asks you whether she's okay. What do you tell Jacklyn?

9. Ms. O'Hara, a 34-year-old computer programmer, is having mild contractions. She is in the 30th week of gestation, and the physician determines that she is experiencing premature labor.

   a.   What agent is the physician likely to prescribe, and how does it work?

   b.   In what position do you place Ms. O'Hara before starting the IV, and why?

   c.   Ms. O'Hara's contractions stop, and she is sent home on maintenance ritodrine therapy. At a follow-up visit, her blood glucose and electrolyte levels are checked. Why?

10. Ms. Jones, a sales associate in a bookstore, is being treated for fertility problems. She is currently on a drug regimen that includes chorionic gonadotropin and Pergonal.

   a.   Why is Ms. Jones taking two fertility agents?

   b.   After the first course of treatment, Ms. Jones does not become pregnant. Describe her next course of treatment.

11. Mrs. Ingalls has been on estrogen therapy for several weeks. During a routine checkup, she sheepishly tells you that she hasn't been able to quit smoking yet. She also mentions that she is going to Aruba for a vacation next month. What patient teaching does Mrs. Ingalls require?

12. Mrs. Simmons, age 33, comes in for her yearly gynecologic examination, and the physician has recommended alendronate (Fosamax), 5 mg daily. Mrs. Simmons experienced early menopause last year and asks you, "Why did the doctor wait until now to start me on estrogen? I didn't need it before."

   a.   What do you explain about the purpose of this medication?

   b.   What risk factors might Mrs. Simmons have to support therapy with alendronate?

Copyright © 2002 by Mosby, Inc. All rights reserved.

Chapter 33

Men's Health Agents

Choose the *best* answer for each of the following.

1. Jack, a member of the college football team, asks his friend's mother, who is a nurse, about taking steroids to help him "beef up" his muscles. Which of the following is true?
   a. There should be no problems as long as he does not exceed the recommended dose.
   b. Long-term use may cause a life-threatening liver condition.
   c. He would need to be careful to watch for excessive weight loss.
   d. These drugs also tend to increase the male's sperm count.

2. In which of the following situations would androgens be prescribed for a woman?
   a. Development of secondary sex characteristics
   b. Postmenopausal osteoporosis prevention
   c. Ovarian cancer
   d. Treatment of endometriosis

3. Samuel will be receiving testosterone therapy for male hypogonadism. The doctor has prescribed Testoderm patches. What does Samuel need to know about the dosage of this medication?
   a. It is applied only on the scrotum
   b. It is never applied to the scrotum.
   c. If the side effects become bothersome, he should stop taking the patch.
   d. It should be applied to a different area of the upper body each day.

4. Rosie will be taking nandrolone as part of the treatment for metastatic breast cancer. Which of the following statements is *not* true regarding therapy with this drug?
   a. She should notify her physician if menstrual irregularities occur.
   b. A low-sodium diet may be recommended if edema occurs.
   c. The strongest dose she can tolerate is needed for optimal therapeutic effect.
   d. Its use is contraindicated if severe cardiac, renal, or liver disease is present.

5. Mr. H. is taking finasteride for the treatment of benign prostatic hypertrophy. His wife, who is 3 months pregnant, is worried about the side effects that may occur with this drug. What is most important to tell them about therapy with this drug?
   a. Gastric upset may be reduced if he takes this on an empty stomach.
   b. They should see therapeutic effects of increased libido and erection in 1 month.
   c. This medication should not even be handled by pregnant women due to its teratogenic effects.
   d. He may experience transient hair loss while on this medication.

CRITICAL THINKING AND APPLICATION

Answer the following questions on a separate sheet of paper.

6. Mr. Michaels has male hypogonadism. He is to receive testosterone cypionate, 75 mg IM, every 2 weeks. You are trying to remember the best means of administering testosterone intramuscularly. A helpful colleague reminds you of its purpose here. You both know that testosterone, when given orally, exhibits poor pharmacokinetics and pharmacodynamics, and you also seem to recall that it is best administered close to the intended site of action for maximum efficacy. Therefore, you reason that it should be injected high in the inner thigh, but not in contact with the groin. A second colleague shrugs and says, "No, no, no. You just use the usual gluteus muscle injection site." Who is right? Where should Mr. Michaels' injection be given?

Copyright © 2002 by Mosby, Inc. All rights reserved.

7. Mr. Michaels is switched to an oral dose form. He expects to get "testosterone pills." However, you remember its poor performance via that route, and you tell him that it will probably not be testosterone itself.

   a. Mr. Michaels is skeptical of switching agents and asks for more explanation. Explain specifically why oral testosterone doesn't work well.

   b. What do you predict Mr. Michaels will receive instead? Discuss potential contraindications that might apply to this patient.

8. Mr. Michaels is administered methyltestosterone buccally. He reports that he gets "tired" of waiting for the buccal tablet to dissolve and asks whether he can swallow or chew it, at least after it is mostly dissolved.

   a. If Mr. Michaels does let it absorb on its own, for the most part, is it acceptable to compromise, for the sake of patient compliance, by letting him chew or swallow the rest?

   b. "And while we're on the subject," Mr. Michaels says, "I'm going on a fishing trip next week. I'd like to not have to bother with the pills. Can we work something out so that I stop temporarily and pick back up with the treatment as soon as I get back?" What do you say?

9. Mr. Olafson has been prescribed finasteride for his benign prostatic hypertrophy. He asks, "How does it work?" You explain that it will cause his prostate to decrease in size and alleviate discomfort.

   a. "No," he says. "You don't understand. I'm not a pharmacist, but I am a chemist. Tell me how it works." Tell him everything you know about how finasteride works.

   b. What are the most important things to include in his patient teaching plan?

10. Mrs. Thiele is taking danazol for endometriosis. Her physician asks you to draw up (and deliver) a patient teaching plan for her. Do so.

11. Mr. A., age 67, has asked the doctor for "help with a private matter." He tells the physician that he would like to try Viagra, "that drug that helps with a certain problem."

   a. What assessment findings may contraindicate the use of sildenafil (Viagra) in Mr. A?

   b. If he was a candidate for therapy with Viagra, what patient teaching should he receive?

Copyright © 2002 by Mosby, Inc. All rights reserved.

Chapter 34

Antihistamines, Decongestants, Antitussives, and Expectorants

Choose the *best* answer for each of the following.

1. When teaching a patient about antihistamine use, which of the following is *not* true?
   a. They are best tolerated when taken with meals.
   b. For dry mouth, the patient can suck on dry candy or chew gum.
   c. The main side effect of antihistamines is drowsiness.
   d. OTC medications are generally safe with antihistamines.

2. Which of the following medications is a nonsedating antihistamine?
   a. loratadine (Claritin)
   b. diphenhydramine (Benadryl)
   c. dimenhydrinate (Dramamine)
   d. meclizine (Antivert)

3. Which agents are considered first-line agents for the treatment of nasal congestion?
   a. Antihistamines such as diphenhydramine
   b. Decongestants such as naphazoline
   c. Antitussives such as dextromethorphan
   d. Expectorants such as guaifenesin

4. Antitussives are used primarily to:
   a. relieve nasal congestion.
   b. thin secretions to ease removal of excessive secretions.
   c. stop the cough reflex when the cough is nonproductive.
   d. suppress productive and nonproductive coughs.

5. Which patient teaching is appropriate for the patient receiving an expectorant?
   a. Avoid fluids for 30 to 35 minutes after the dose.
   b. Force fluids, unless contraindicated, to aid in expectoration of sputum.
   c. Avoid driving or operating heavy machinery while on this medication.
   d. Patients should expect their secretions to become thicker.

CRITICAL THINKING AND APPLICATION

Answer the following questions on a separate sheet of paper.

6. Why are H_1 blockers most beneficial when given early in a reaction?

7. Do the traditional antihistamines have any advantages over the newer, nonsedating antihistamines? Explain your answer.

8. James, a 35-year-old electrician, is seen in the ER with a rash on his arms and hands that appeared after he was working in his yard. You suspect that the physician will prescribe topical diphenhydramine, but during the nursing assessment, James tells you that he has diabetes.

   a. How does James's diabetes affect his possible treatment with diphenhydramine?

   b. If James does receive a topical diphenhydramine, what other agent might be found in combination with it?

   c. What are some other indications for diphenhydramine?

Copyright © 2002 by Mosby, Inc. All rights reserved.

9. Mrs. Ling was seen in the office several days ago with a common cold. She has been on decongestant therapy with naphazoline since that time. Today she calls to say, "I thought I was getting over this, but suddenly my nose is more stuffed up than ever." Does Mrs. Ling possibly need a stronger dosage of the decongestant? Explain your answer.

10. Keith has been using a topical nasal decongestant for the past few days. He calls the physician's office to report that he is feeling nervous and dizzy and that his heart seems to be racing. What might be the cause of Keith's symptoms?

11. How does benzonatate differ from other antitussive agents in its mechanism of action? What about in its drug interaction profile?

12. One day you encounter your neighbor Irene as you are returning home from work. She is on her way to the drugstore, she tells you, because she has been experiencing a nonproductive cough and wants to get "a cough medicine to loosen things up." You recall Irene mentioning a few months ago that she has problems with her thyroid. Do you wish Irene good luck and continue on your way? Explain your answer.

13. Lisa is a 5-year-old patient with bronchitis accompanied by a nonproductive cough. The physician has prescribed Robitussin for the cough. Lisa's father tells you that his 11-year-old son was prescribed Robitussin A-C several months ago for a severe cough. He asks you whether his son's cough medicine would help Lisa since "there is plenty left in the bottle." What do you tell him?

Copyright © 2002 by Mosby, Inc. All rights reserved.

Chapter 35

Bronchodilators and Other Respiratory Agents

Choose the *best* answer for each of the following.

1. Frequent use of bronchodilators may cause all the following side effects *except*:
   a. blurred vision.
   b. increased heart rate.
   c. nervousness.
   d. tremors.

2. Maggie will be taking cromolyn sodium inhalers to treat her asthma. It is important to teach her which of the following regarding this medication?
   a. If a dose is missed, she may take a double dose to maintain blood levels.
   b. In order to maintain the inhaled medication's effect, she should not gargle or rinse her mouth after using the inhaler.
   c. She should take this inhaler at the first sign of bronchospasm.
   d. Administer the medication consistently, and be aware that up to 4 weeks may be needed to see therapeutic effects.

3. Which drug acts by blocking leukotrienes, thus reducing inflammation in the lungs?
   a. albuterol (Proventil)
   b. cromolyn (Intal)
   c. theophylline (Theo-Dur)
   d. zafirlukast (Accolate)

4. Which drug is used for status asthmaticus in patients who have not responded to epinephrine?
   a. albuterol (Proventil)
   b. aminophylline
   c. theophylline (Theo-Dur)
   d. montelukast (Singulair)

5. When testing an MDI canister to estimate whether it is empty, the inhaler canister (not the mouthpiece) is dropped into a container that is wider and longer than the inhaler and filled up to three-quarters full with water. Which indicates that the inhaler canister is nearly empty?
   a. The canister drops to the bottom of the water container and lies on its side.
   b. The canister drops to the bottom of the water container, but the bottom of the canister points upward.
   c. The canister floats on top of the water line.
   d. The canister floats halfway in the water, and halfway out of the water.

CRITICAL THINKING AND APPLICATION

Answer the following questions on a separate sheet of paper.

6. Describe briefly how idiopathic asthma differs from allergic asthma.

7. Ms. Ward has been admitted to the hospital with status asthmaticus. A nursing assessment reveals that she has a history of alcoholism and seizures. The physician prescribes aminophylline IV. Later, a student nurse, who was present in Ms. Ward's room, approaches you and says, "Last week that same doctor gave epinephrine to a patient having an asthma attack. Why not now?" What do you say?

8. Yuri has left-sided heart failure. What agent might be helpful, and how will it work in Yuri's case?

Copyright © 2002 by Mosby, Inc. All rights reserved.

9. Tom, a 70-year-old retiree who smoked for 40 years, has been diagnosed with COPD; his treatment will include theophylline. After a few weeks, Tom tells you that he is experiencing nausea and "bad heartburn at night." The laboratory studies show the level of theophylline in his blood to be 30 µg/ml. What might be wrong with Tom, and how can it be corrected?

10. Willie is a 9-year-old boy who is brought to the ER by his aunt because he is having an acute asthma attack. The physician orders epinephrine SC. How do you calculate the dosage for Willie?

11. Sylvia has come to the clinic today complaining of nausea, palpitations, and anxiety. She says that her heart feels "as if it's going to fly out of my chest." Physical examination confirms an increased heart rate. Sylvia's records indicate that she has asthma for which she uses an albuterol inhaler. What do you suspect might be wrong with Sylvia, and what do you advise her?

12. Mrs. Voss, a 65-year-old office manager, has arthritis, glaucoma, and emphysema. The physician is planning prophylactic treatment.

    a. What three types of agents might be considered for prophylactic treatment of a patient with COPD?

    b. What factor must the physician keep in mind when determining the best agent for Mrs. Voss?

13. Several months ago the physician prescribed an orally administered corticosteroid for Mr. Zoller, who has chronic bronchial asthma.

    a. What are the disadvantages of administering the corticosteroids orally?

    b. Today the physician adds Beclovent to Mr. Zoller's drug regimen and also reduces the dosage of the oral corticosteroid. Is that safe?

14. Mr. Wells, a 30-year-old mail carrier, has asthma that is exacerbated by cold weather. He has had several asthma attacks while walking his mail route.

    a. What type of agent would be helpful for Mr. Wells, and how will it probably be administered?

    b. What problem might occur during delivery of the drug, and how should it be handled?

    c. What patient teaching will you stress for Mr. Wells?

15. Sam is a 10-year-old girl who is to be treated with theophylline for her asthma.

    a. What particular effect will have to be watched for, and why?

    b. Sam's mother asks whether she can crush the tablets to make them easier for Sam to swallow. Is that advisable?

16. Ms. Weaver takes an oral corticosteroid as part of the therapy for her chronic asthma. During an office visit for treatment following a fall, Ms. Weaver mentions that she "started back on the pill" a few weeks ago. She also comments that she is "getting fat," having gained 6 pounds in less than 2 weeks during the holidays. What do you do?

Copyright © 2002 by Mosby, Inc. All rights reserved.

Chapter 36

Antibiotics

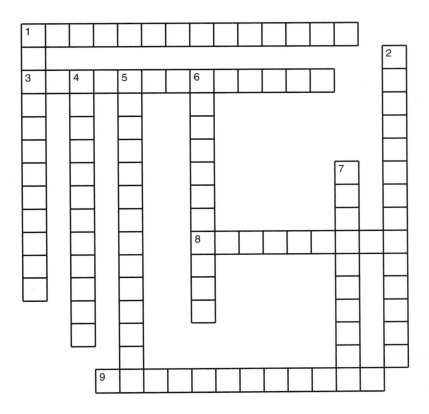

Across

1. Antibiotics that inhibit the growth of bacteria.
3. The classification for the drug cefazolin.
8. The classification for the drug erythromycin.
9. The classification for the drug doxycycline.

Down

1. Antibiotics that kill bacteria.
2. An infection that occurs during antimicrobial treatment for another infection and results in overgrowth of a nonsusceptible organism.
4. Antibiotics taken before exposure to an infectious organism in an effort to prevent the development of infection.
5. The classification for the drug amikacin.
6. The classification for the drug sulfisoxazole.
7. An antibiotic derived from a fungus, or mold, often seen on bread or fruit.

Copyright © 2002 by Mosby, Inc. All rights reserved.

Choose the *best* answer for each of the following.

1. A drug interaction occurs with penicillins and which of the following?
   a. Alcohol
   b. Anticonvulsants
   c. digoxin
   d. NSAIDs

2. Specific nursing interventions for the patient taking sulfonamides include all of the following *except*:
   a. obtaining a culture and sensitivity before beginning the antibiotic.
   b. assessing for allergic reaction.
   c. monitoring urinary output.
   d. restricting oral fluids.

3. Which of the following would *not* be included in the patient teaching for the patient receiving penicillin antibiotic therapy?
   a. Use antibiotics from previous prescriptions.
   b. Take the antibiotic for the length of time prescribed.
   c. Take oral forms with 6 to 8 ounces of water to improve absorption.
   d. Report sore throat, fever, or joint pain to the physician immediately.

4. Recommendations for taking tetracycline would include:
   a. taking it with milk.
   b. taking it with 8 ounces of water.
   c. taking it 30 minutes before taking iron preparations.
   d. using an antacid to decrease discomfort.

5. Patients with a history of sensitivity to which of the following products should *not* be given cephalosporins?
   a. Antihypertensives
   b. Thiazide diuretics
   c. Penicillins
   d. Antacids

6. Patients receiving aminglycosides must be monitored for tinnitus, which may indicate:
   a. cardiotoxicity.
   b. hepatotoxicity.
   c. ototoxicity.
   d. nephrotoxicity.

CRITICAL THINKING AND APPLICATION

Answer the following questions on a separate sheet of paper.

7. Mr. Renville, a 50-year-old banker, is scheduled for colorectal surgery tomorrow. The surgeon is planning to administer a prophylactic antibiotic. What agent is frequently used for this purpose, and why?

8. Sean is a 19-year-old college freshman who has been diagnosed with gonorrhea. The physician has prescribed doxycycline therapy. During your nursing assessment, you and Sean discuss his diet, which includes "lots of meat, milk, and veggies." Sean also tells you that he jogs frequently and is a member of the tennis team.

   a. In addition to instruction about sexually transmitted diseases, what patient teaching does Sean require?

   b. A few days later Sean calls and complains of an upset stomach and diarrhea. What do you suspect might be wrong with Sean?

9. Virgil has been admitted to your unit and placed on aminoglycoside therapy.

   a. What two serious toxicities will you monitor for, what are their symptoms, and how can they be prevented?

   b. The physician adds penicillin to Virgil's drug regimen. Why?

Copyright © 2002 by Mosby, Inc. All rights reserved.

Chapter 37

Antiviral Agents

Choose the *best* answer for each of the following.

1. Acyclovir is considered the drug of choice for:
   a. cytomegalovirus.
   b. HIV.
   c. RSV.
   d. varicella-zoster.

2. Amantadine is only active against:
   a. cytomegalovirus.
   b. influenza A.
   c. HSV-2.
   d. varicella-zoster.

3. What would be a contraindication to the use of foscarnet?
   a. Renal toxicity
   b. CMV retinitis
   c. Asthma
   d. Immunosuppression

4. Amantadine would be used in which of the following patients?
   a. A 29-year-old male who is HIV-positive
   b. A 22-year-old female, who is in her 8th month of pregnancy and HIV-positive
   c. As prophylaxis for influenza A virus in a heart transplant patient
   d. As prophylaxis for influenza B in elderly patients

5. Which of the following is an indication for the use of oseltamivir (Tamiflu)?
   a. Prevention of infection after exposure to influenza types A and B
   b. Reduction of the duration of the flu by several days in adults
   c. Treatment of topical herpes simplex infections
   d. Reduction of the severity of shingles symptoms

CRITICAL THINKING AND APPLICATION

Answer the following questions on a separate sheet of paper.

6. Why are so few antiviral agents available? Why are viruses so difficult to kill?

7. Amy is 12 weeks into her pregnancy when she discovers she is HIV-positive. Amy is very upset and says, "I won't live long enough to have this baby. We're both going to die." Is it possible to treat Amy and/or the fetus? Explain your answer.

8. Bailey, a 53-year-old teacher with osteoporosis, has shingles.

   a. What agent do you expect the physician to prescribe?

   b. What instructions will you give Bailey regarding any dietary considerations?

   c. Several months later, Bailey calls the office to say that her symptoms have returned. What action do you expect to be taken now?

101

Copyright © 2002 by Mosby, Inc. All rights reserved.

9. Cary, a 30-year-old stockbroker, has been diagnosed with genital herpes simplex. The physician has prescribed topical Zovirax.

    a.   What patient teaching do you provide to Cary regarding administration of this agent?

    b.   Cary asks you how long it will take for the Zovirax to cure his herpes. What is your reply?

    c.   What else should you discuss with Cary, who is single?

10. Brenda is a 5-year-old who has bronchopneumonia caused by RSV.

    a.   What antiviral agent is used to treat RSV?

    b.   Brenda's mother wonders whether the treatment will be completed before Brenda's birthday, which is just 2 weeks away. What do you tell her?

11. Mr. Castelli, an inpatient, has developed herpes simplex keratoconjunctivitis. The physician has prescribed Viroptic, and you are reviewing the administration technique with a new nurse.

    a.   What basic but vital information do you discuss?

    b.   What side/adverse effects will you tell the nurse to monitor for?

    c.   Mr. Castelli tells you that he "can't stand" having medication put in his eyes and wants to know whether there's a tablet or capsule he can take. What do you tell him?

12. Eduardo, a 25-year-old translator, has AIDS. He was treated with AZT for several months, but now the physician has switched him to didanosine powder.

    a.   What frequently is the reason that patients are switched from AZT to another anti-HIV agent?

    b.   What instructions do you give Eduardo regarding administration of the didanosine?

    c.   Should Eduardo discontinue the antacid he has been taking? Explain your answer.

13. You overhear a co-worker explaining to a student nurse the procedure for administering acyclovir IV. After diluting the acyclovir in sterile water, your co-worker says, "We'll administer this over at least an hour." Should you intervene? Explain your answer.

Copyright © 2002 by Mosby, Inc. All rights reserved.

Chapter 38

Antitubercular Agents

_____

Choose the *best* answer for each of the following.

1. During INH therapy, what laboratory work would be monitored closely?
   a. Liver enzymes
   b. Hct/Hgb
   c. Creatinine
   d. Platelet count

2. What would you expect to include in the teaching plan for a patient who is taking INH?
   a. Urine and saliva may be reddish-orange in color.
   b. Pyridoxine may be needed to prevent neurotoxicity.
   c. Injection sites should be rotated daily.
   d. Take medications with an antacid to reduce gastric distress.

3. Patients who are in the initial period of treatment for tuberculosis need to be taught all the following *except*:
   a. to wash their hands and cover their mouth when coughing or sneezing to reduce the spread of TB.
   b. to throw away dirty tissues with care.
   c. to be sure to get adequate rest, nutrition, and relaxation.
   d. that medication doses may be skipped occasionally if gastric distress occurs.

4. Drug therapy as the treatment for active tuberculosis may need to last up to:
   a. 6 months.
   b. 12 months.
   c. 24 months.
   d. a lifetime.

5. Why are multiple medications used in the drug regimen for tuberculosis?
   a. It reduces the possibility of the organism becoming drug-resistant.
   b. It ensures a 99% cure of the disease.
   c. Starting drug therapy early on will reduce symptoms immediately.
   d. Patient compliance is better with multiple medications.

CRITICAL THINKING AND APPLICATION

Answer the following questions on a separate sheet of paper.

6. Diane, a 33-year-old proofreader, has been prescribed prophylactic isoniazid treatment.

   a. What laboratory studies should be performed before the start of therapy? Why?

   b. After Diane has taken the isoniazid for 2 months, the physician significantly reduces her dosage of the drug. Why might that be?

Copyright © 2002 by Mosby, Inc. All rights reserved.

7. Ms. Innes is undergoing antitubercular therapy that includes streptomycin.

   a. How is streptomycin administered?

   b. What side/adverse effects will you monitor for?

   c. Ms. Innes takes an oral contraceptive. Is that a concern with Ms. Innes's streptomycin therapy? Explain your answer.

8. Why would an eye examination be performed before instituting antitubercular therapy?

9. George, a 73-year-old retired plant foreman, has been diagnosed with TB. Nursing assessment reveals a history of gout and diabetes.

   a. What considerations will the physician keep in mind when deciding on a first-line agent for George?

   b. The physician prescribes INH. What important instructions do you give George, who is also diabetic?

10. Mr. Fiore, a 42-year-old marketing executive, is on antitubercular therapy. During his first follow-up visit, he is evasive when you ask him about his compliance with his therapy. He does tell you that he has been very busy lately, entertaining various clients "at everything from cocktail parties to big sit-down dinners."

   a. What issues should you discuss with Mr. Fiore?

   b. Several weeks later, Mr. Fiore returns for another follow-up visit. On examination, you see no apparent signs of the TB. How can Mr. Fiore's therapeutic response be confirmed?

11. Frannie is a homeless 68-year-old woman who lives in a shelter some of the time. She was diagnosed at the community health clinic with TB, and antitubercular therapy has been instituted.

   a. What patient education issues are of particular concern in Frannie's case?

   b. Frannie is staying at the shelter and seems to be handling her medication regimen well, but one day she comes by the clinic to tell you that she is afraid the medication may be bad for her. "Whenever I go to the bathroom, everything is orange," she says. What do you suppose is wrong, and what do you tell Frannie?

Copyright © 2002 by Mosby, Inc. All rights reserved.

Chapter 39

Antifungal Agents

Match each definition with its corresponding term.

1. _____ Single-celled fungi that reproduce by budding.

2. _____ One of the four major groups of antifungal agents, including amphotericin B and nystatin.

3. _____ A very large, diverse group of eukaryotic, thallus-forming microorganisms that require an external carbon source.

4. _____ One of the four major groups of antifungal agents, including ketoconazole, miconazole, and clotrimazole.

5. _____ A term for yeast infection of the mouth.

6. _____ One of the four major groups of antifungals; acts by preventing susceptible fungi from reproducing.

7. _____ The earliest antifungal agent.

8. _____ An antifungal agent commonly used for candidal diaper rash.

9. _____ An infection caused by fungi.

10. _____ Multicellular fungi characterized by long, branching filaments called hyphae, which entwine to form a mycelium.

a. Thrush

b. Molds

c. griseofulvin

d. Mycosis

e. Polyenes

f. Fungi

g. Imidazoles

h. amphotericin B

i. nystatin

j. Yeast

Choose the *best* answer for each of the following.

11. Which of the following would be used to treat thrush in an infant?
    a. amphotericin B
    b. fluconazole
    c. nystatin
    d. miconazole

12. Which of the following are side effects of amphotericin B infusions?
    a. Anorexia, abdominal cramps, and diarrhea
    b. Fever, chills, and malaise
    c. Rash, urticaria, and angioedema
    d. Drowsiness, confusion, and fatigue

13. Women who begin to menstruate while taking vaginal medications for vaginal infections should:
    a. stop the medication until the menstrual flow has stopped.
    b. take the medication at night only.
    c. stop the medication for 3 days, then resume.
    d. continue to take the medication.

14. Which medication is often used as a 1-day dose treatment of vaginal candidiasis?
    a. ketoconazole
    b. fluconazole
    c. griseofulvin
    d. imidazole

105

Copyright © 2002 by Mosby, Inc. All rights reserved.

15. Which is the agent of choice for treatment of many severe systemic fungal infections?
    a. amphotericin B
    b. fluconazole
    c. griseofulvin
    d. flucytosine

CRITICAL THINKING AND APPLICATION

Answer the following questions on a separate sheet of paper.

16. Why are there so few oral and parenteral agents to treat mycotic infections?

17. Mr. Kim has been diagnosed with cryptococcal meningitis, and the physician has prescribed Diflucan.

    a. Why did the physician choose this agent rather than the other imidazoles?

    b. Mr. Kim's CSF culture eventually comes back negative. When he hears the good news, he says, "Great! I'm tired of taking this medicine." What is your response?

18. The physician is planning IV amphotericin B therapy for James.

    a. What guidelines do you follow in diluting the agent?

    b. What side effects do you expect James to experience?

    c. Should you stop the infusion if those effects occur? Explain your answer.

19. Lewis has a severe ringworm infection for which the physician has prescribed griseofulvin. During your nursing assessment, Lewis tells you that he hopes the infection will clear up soon, because he is going on a cruise ship in 2 weeks and he plans to "party every night!" What patient teaching issues should you discuss with Lewis?

Copyright © 2002 by Mosby, Inc. All rights reserved.

Chapter 40

Antimalarial, Antiprotozoal, and Antihelmintic Agents

Choose the *best* answer for each of the following.

1. Which of the following contraindications should be assessed in a patient before beginning antiprotozoal therapy?
   a. Underlying renal, cardiac, thyroid, or liver disease and pregnancy
   b. Porphyria and G6PD deficiency
   c. Glaucoma, cataracts, anemia, and petechiae
   d. Constipation, gastritis, and lactose intolerance

2. The patient taking thiabendazole should be warned about which possible side effect?
   a. Reddish-orange urine
   b. Urine with an asparagus-like odor
   c. A metallic taste in the mouth
   d. Severe halitosis

3. Why would a sulfonamide or tetracycline be given with quinine therapy in mild cases of malaria?
   a. The antibiotic treats bacterial infections that accompany malaria.
   b. The antibiotic reduces the severe side effects of quinine.
   c. These antibiotics have a synergistic effect with quinine.
   d. The antibiotic therapy is also needed to kill the parasite that causes malaria.

4. Which agent is used mainly for the management of *Pneumocystis carinii* pneumonia?
   a. metronidazole
   b. pentamidine
   c. primaquine
   d. pyrantel

5. Which of the following is true regarding patients receiving anthelmintic therapy?
   a. The medication can be stopped once symptoms disappear.
   b. The medication must be taken exactly as ordered for the length of time ordered.
   c. Anthelmintics are broad in their actions and can be substituted easily if one medication is not well-tolerated.
   d. Anthelmintics are more effective in their parenteral forms.

CRITICAL THINKING AND APPLICATION

Answer the following questions on a separate sheet of paper.

6. Professor Henson has just returned from a research sabbatical in Africa, where she did not adequately protect herself from mosquito exposure; thus, she has contracted malaria. What kind of parasite causes malaria? Which drug is recommended if the parasite is in the exoerythrocytic phase of development? What exactly is the exoerythrocytic phase?

7. Professor Henson's physician would like to prescribe the drug you identified in your answer to question 6. You should assess this patient for which kind of contraindications?

Copyright © 2002 by Mosby, Inc. All rights reserved.

8. Professor Henson's husband, who accompanied her on her trip, has even more recently begun to develop signs of malaria. He is given chloroquine, a 4-aminoquinoline derivative. However, unlike his wife, Mr. Henson shows no sign of seeing his symptoms lessen. His strain of malaria appears to be chloroquine-resistant. What alternative(s) can you suggest for Mr. Henson?

9. The medical clinic in which you work has a full waiting room this morning. Patient A is being seen for an intestinal disorder that he acquired after swimming in Lake Michigan. Patient B is an AIDS patient who is showing early signs of pneumonia. Patient C is being treated and evaluated on a regular basis for a sexually transmitted disease. Here's your challenge: All three patients have something in common regarding the etiologies of their disorders. Discern what that could be. Second, based on that commonality, predict what disorder, of those discussed in this chapter, each patient might have. (Hint: One patient has giardiasis, but we're not saying who.) Third, select a drug you feel the physician is likely to prescribe for each patient.

10. Mr. Aubrey has been diagnosed with schistosomiasis; his physician prescribes oxamniquine therapy. The physician has explained to Mr. Aubrey the drug's mechanism of action. Mr. Aubrey jokes to you that perhaps he ought to "drink plenty of milk now to help the medication do its job." Given what you know about oxamniquine's mechanism of action, explain what might lead Mr. Aubrey to say this.

Copyright © 2002 by Mosby, Inc. All rights reserved.

Chapter 41

Antiseptic and Disinfectant Agents

CRITICAL THINKING CROSSWORD

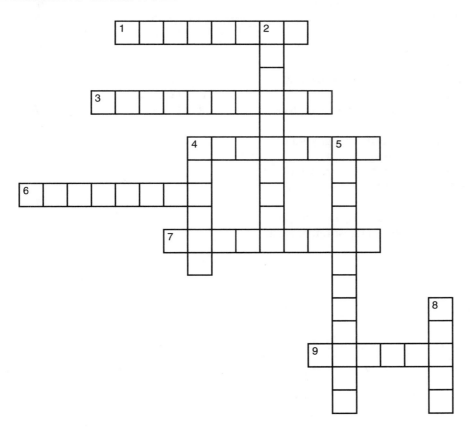

Across

1. A surface-active agent.
3. An infection acquired at least 72 hours after hospitalization.
4. The classification of Cidex.
6. An iodine agent widely used as an antiseptic.
7. Chlorhexidine gluconate.
9. A sodium hypochlorite solution.

Down

2. A substance that inhibits the growth and reproduction of microorganisms without necessarily killing them.
4. An acid used in a 5% solution for killing microorganisms.
5. A chemical applied to nonliving objects to destroy microorganisms.
8. An example of a phenolic compound.

Copyright © 2002 by Mosby, Inc. All rights reserved.

Choose the *best* answer for each of the following.

1. Which of the following statements about nosocomial infections is *not* true?
   a. They are contracted in the home or community.
   b. They are contracted in a hospital or institution.
   c. They are more difficult to treat.
   d. The organisms that cause these infections are more virulent.

2. Which statement accurately describes the action of antiseptics?
   a. They are used to kill organisms on nonliving objects.
   b. They are used to kill organisms on living tissue.
   c. They are used to prevent the growth of organisms on nonliving objects.
   d. They are used to inhibit the growth of organisms on living tissue.

3. Which concentration of isopropanol (isopropyl alcohol) is most effective against microorganisms?
   a. 5%
   b. 25%
   c. 50%
   d. 70%

4. Before using Betadine solution as a skin prep for surgery, you should ask the patient about allergies to which substance?
   a. Shellfish
   b. Penicillin
   c. Mercury
   d. Milk

5. If a patient is allergic to povidone-iodine, which agent may be used instead as a surgical scrub?
   a. Acetic acid
   b. Hibiclens
   c. Gentian violet
   d. Phenol

Copyright © 2002 by Mosby, Inc. All rights reserved.

Chapter 42

Antiinflammatory, Antirheumatoid, and Related Agents

Choose the *best* answer for each of the following.

1. A common side effect of NSAID therapy is:
   a. diarrhea.
   b. GI distress.
   c. hypotension.
   d. palpitations.

2. Emily, age 13, has the flu, and her mother is concerned about her fever of 103° F. Which medication should be used to treat Emily's fever?
   a. aspirin
   b. acetaminophen
   c. indomethacin
   d. naproxen

3. Henry is being treated with allopurinol for an acute flare-up of gout. All of the following should be included in a teaching plan for Henry *except*:
   a. avoiding alcohol and caffeine.
   b. taking the medication with meals to prevent GI symptoms.
   c. taking the medication on an empty stomach to improve absorption.
   d. increasing fluid intake up to 3 to 4 L per day.

4. Contraindications for the use of NSAIDs include:
   a. pericarditis.
   b. osteoarthritis.
   c. bleeding disorders.
   d. juvenile rheumatoid arthritis

5. The patient receiving gold injections as treatment for arthritis should be told:
   a. that injections will be given via the intravenous route.
   b. that the medication is more effective if fluids are restricted.
   c. to expect relief from symptoms in a few days.
   d. that relief from symptoms may take up to 3 to 4 months.

CRITICAL THINKING AND APPLICATION

Answer the following questions on a separate sheet of paper.

6. Ms. Bailey is brought into the ER exhibiting the following symptoms: tinnitus, hearing loss, dimming vision, and dizziness. She is also very thirsty and sweating profusely. Drinking water only exacerbates her GI distress, which includes forceful, frequent vomiting. On examination you discover that she has an increased heart rate and is suffering some confusion. At first she appears drowsy and then begins to hyperventilate. You suspect salicylism, but your colleague says, "No, this is acute salicylate intoxication." If he is right? How was he able to tell? What causes each?

7. Ms. Bailey turns out to have acute toxicity stemming from a salicylate overdose. Describe an appropriate treatment plan.

8. Mr. Chesney presents with symptoms that are similar to Ms. Bailey's but not as extensive. He is experiencing drowsiness, mental confusion, numbness, and disorientation. His behavior is aggressive, with seizures, nausea and vomiting, and GI bleeding. What is wrong? What would you expect if it were allowed to progress?

111

Copyright © 2002 by Mosby, Inc. All rights reserved.

9. How will Mr. Chesney's treatment differ from Mrs. Bailey's?

10. Mr. Henry has come to the clinic complaining of a severe flare-up of his gout. He tells you that he does not take his medicine on a regular basis because it "kills" his stomach. He also says he hates to take medicine but hates the gout more. He has a prescription for allopurinol and a follow-up appointment for next week. What patient teaching does Mr. Henry need?

Copyright © 2002 by Mosby, Inc. All rights reserved.

Chapter 43

Immunosuppressant Agents

Choose the *best* answer for each of the following.

1. The major risk factor for patients on immuno-suppressants is:
   a. severe hypotension with potential renal failure.
   b. an increased susceptibility to opportunistic infections.
   c. decreased platelet aggregation.
   d. increased bleeding tendencies.

2. Which agent is used to treat organ rejection once rejection of a transplanted organ is under-way?
   a. azathioprine
   b. cyclosporine
   c. muromonab-CD3
   d. tacrolimus

3. Which may cause an increase in the bioavail-ability of cyclosporine when taken together?
   a. Dairy products
   b. Orange juice
   c. Grapefruit juice
   d. Red wines

4. When taking oral doses of immunosuppres-sants, the patient should take them:
   a. with food to minimize GI upset.
   b. on an empty stomach to increase absorp-tion rates.
   c. only when side effects are tolerable.
   d. with antacids.

5. Patients taking immunosuppressants should be told all the following *except*:
   a. to avoid crowds to minimize the risk of infection.
   b. to report any fever, sore throat, chills or joint pain.
   c. that lifelong therapy is indicated with organ transplantation.
   d. to expect to take these drugs for up to 1 year after an organ transplant.

CRITICAL THINKING AND APPLICATION

Answer the following questions on a separate sheet of paper.

6. Mrs. Flick is about to undergo heart transplant surgery. The physician plans to begin her on cyclosporine therapy.

   a. Mrs. Flick asks you why.

   b. Describe the laboratory studies to be performed and documented. How often should they be done? What purpose do they serve?

7. Mrs. Flick is convinced that the cyclosporine is upsetting her stomach.

   a. What can you say?

   b. Three days before her surgery, an oral antifungal is added to Mrs. Flick's regimen. "Why?" she says, "Is this related to my stomach upset?"

113

Copyright © 2002 by Mosby, Inc. All rights reserved.

8. Mrs. Flick's roommate, Tess, is hoping to have a renal transplant. She is taking muromonab-CD3, IV, 5 mg/day in a single bolus. On her second day, she begins to exhibit chest pain, dyspnea, and wheezing. Her leukocyte count is 4000/mm^3. What is happening? What might you suggest?

9. Tess is found to be an excellent candidate for a renal transplant; the surgery will take place in a couple of days. She is switched to azathioprine, PO, 3.5 mg/kg/day. Why?

Copyright © 2002 by Mosby, Inc. All rights reserved.

Chapter 44

Immunizing Agents

1. Complete the following chart by filling in all missing information.

Agent	Active or Passive?	Purpose
a.	b.	Chicken pox
Hib	c.	d.
e.	Active	Hepatitis B virus prophylaxis
f.	g.	Postpartum antibody suppression
BCG vaccine	h.	i.
DTaP	j.	k.
Tetanus immune globulin-TIG	l.	m.
Td	n.	o.

Choose the *best* answer for each of the following.

2. The immunity that is passed from a mother to her nursing infant through antibodies in breast milk is called:
   a. artificially acquired passive immunity.
   b. naturally acquired passive immunity.
   c. active immunity.
   d. immune globulins.

3. Which of the following contain substances that trigger the formation of antibodies against specific pathogens?
   a. Antivenins
   b. Serums
   c. Toxoids
   d. Vaccines

4. Which preparation confers long-lasting immunity against a particular pathogen?
   a. Poliovirus vaccine, live oral
   b. Immune globulin IV
   c. Rh_o immune globulin
   d. Black widow spider antivenin

5. Christie, the mother of 6-month-old Jack, says that the last time he received a DtaP the injection site on his leg was warm, slightly swollen, and red. You are preparing another dose of the vaccine. You should:
   a. explain that these effects can be expected and give the medication.
   b. give half the prescribed dose this week and the other half next week if tolerated well.
   c. skip the dose and notify the physician.
   d. wait 6 months and then administer the dose.

6. Goldie has been stuck by a used needle while starting an IV. Which preparation is used as prophylaxis against disease after exposure to blood and body fluids?
   a. Hib vaccine
   b. $Rh_0(D)$ immune globulin
   c. hepatitis B immune globulin
   d. hepatitis antitoxin

Copyright © 2002 by Mosby, Inc. All rights reserved.

CRITICAL THINKING AND APPLICATION

Answer the following questions on a separate sheet of paper.

7. Jim, a cabinetmaker, was cut by a woodworking tool and came to the clinic for stitches. When the nurse asked him about his tetanus vaccination history, he said, "I have no idea when my last tetanus shot was—I thought once I had all the shots for school that I was set for life! I don't need any more." What do you explain to Jim?

8. Mrs. James, an 82-year-old widow, is in the office for a follow-up appointment to evaluate her emphysema. The physician recommends that she have an influenza virus vaccine. As you prepare the injection, Mrs. James says, "I had a flu shot last year—why do I need another one this year?" What is your explanation to her?

9. Mr. Smythe brings his toddler, Carl, in for a 12-month well-child check. Before giving the MMR injection, what side effects do you tell Mr. Smythe to watch for in Carl's response to the immunization? What can be done to relieve these side effects?

Copyright © 2002 by Mosby, Inc. All rights reserved.

Chapter 45

Antineoplastic Agents

CRITICAL THINKING CROSSWORD

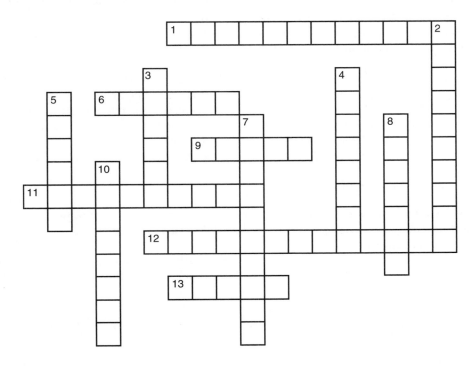

Across

1. Mr. Harris's physician explains that some of the agents he is a candidate for have two reactive alkyl groups to work on two DNA molecules. Thus, they are _____ agents.
6. Mr. Kilpatrick's physician is not surprised to find that cisplatin is killing the cells of his stomach, resulting in nausea and vomiting; he is not surprised, but he is disappointed to find that cisplatin is displaying such a strong _____ potential in this patient.
9. Mr. Heath is prescribed methotrexate. He asks for a full description of its mechanism of action, so you explain how it will inhibit dihydrofolic reductase from converting _____ acid to a reduced folate, thus ultimately preventing synthesis of DNA and cell reproduction. The end result, you explain, is that the cell will die.
11. Ms. Patchett had a biopsy done on the same day as Ms. Lilliankamp (from 3 Down); however, her results are just the opposite of Ms.

Lilliankamp's, meaning that her lump is a(n) _____.

12. Mr. Bronte has just been through a series of chemotherapeutic treatments when he discovers that the antineoplastic agent has leaked into surrounding tissues; in other words, _____ of the agent has occurred.
13. Mr. Cunningham is very interested in his chemotherapeutic process. As you are discussing a drug's action, he hears you use the term _____, and he asks you what it means. You explain that this refers to the time frame in which this particular agent will kill bone marrow cells.

Down

2. Mr. Kellogg has been treated with methotrexate for its folate-antagonistic properties. Now, however, he seems to be experiencing a toxicity reaction. What treatment medium can you suggest to reverse this?

Copyright © 2002 by Mosby, Inc. All rights reserved.

3. Ms. Lilliankamp recently had a biopsy for a lump near her breast. After waiting several days, her physician calls and tells her that the lump is noncancerous and therefore not an immediate threat to life. She is pleased to hear, then, that it is _____.

4. Ms. Hart has a malignant neoplasm of the blood-forming tissues. Her bone marrow is being rapidly replaced with proliferating leukocyte precursors; she also has abnormal numbers (and forms) of immature white cells in her circulation, and even her lymph nodes, spleen, and liver are being infiltrated. Ms. Hart apparently has _____.

5. Mr. Harris is told that his cancer has metastasized. You explain to him that this means it has _____.

7. Mr. Harris has been diagnosed with chronic lymphocytic leukemia; Ms. Fehrers has multiple myeloma. Both patients will need treat-

ment with an agent that can generate a reaction called _____, which, occurring with a cellular constituent such as DNA, will interfere with the cancer's mitosis and cell division.

8. Mr. Kilpatrick, who has testicular cancer, is receiving cisplatin because of its ability to interfere with the process of cancerous cell reproduction, which, unabated, would result in the formation of two genetically identical daughter cancer cells containing the diploid number of chromosomes needed for its proliferation. In other words, you explain, cisplatin will interfere with the cancer's _____ and cell division.

10. Ms. Fehrers has subsequently been given her first chemotherapy treatment. However, it soon becomes apparent that the side effects she is experiencing prevent her from being given doses that will be high enough to be effective. These are dose-_____ side effects.

Choose the *best* answer for each of the following.

1. General adverse effects of antineoplastic drugs include all of the following *except*:
   a. bone marrow suppression.
   b. infertility.
   c. stomatitis.
   d. urinary retention.

2. Leucovorin is required as a rescue for normal cells with administration of high doses of:
   a. bleomycin.
   b. cisplatin.
   c. methotrexate.
   d. dactinomycin.

3. Tumors that respond best to chemotherapy are those with:
   a. long doubling times.
   b. very large mass.
   c. high-growth fraction.
   d. low-growth fraction.

4. A cell-cycle nonspecific (CCNS) agent effective in inhibiting any phase of the cancer cell cycle is:
   a. methotrexate (antimetabolite).
   b. Cytoxan (alkylating agent).
   c. 5-fluorouracil (5-FU).
   d. vincristine.

5. Combinations of chemotherapeutic agents are frequently used today in order to:
   a. prevent drug resistance.
   b. reduce the incidence of side effects.

   c. decrease the cost of treatment.
   d. reduce treatment time.

6. If extravasation of a neoplastic agents occurs, which of the following actions should *not* be taken?
   a. Remove the IV catheter immediately.
   b. Stop the agent but leave in the IV tube.
   c. Aspirate residual drug or blood from the tube if possible.
   d. Administer the appropriate antidote.

7. Symptoms of stomatitis include:
   a. indigestion and heartburn.
   b. white patches and ulcerations of the mouth.
   c. severe vomiting and anorexia.
   d. diarrhea and perianal irritation.

8. Which cytotoxic antibiotic is used to treat solid tumors?
   a. Taxol
   b. vincristine
   c. Cytoxan
   d. bleomycin

9. All of the following are considered dose-limiting side effects of antineoplastic therapy except:
   a. pain.
   b. hair loss.
   c. nausea and vomiting.
   d. myelosuppression.

Copyright © 2002 by Mosby, Inc. All rights reserved.

Chapter 46

Biologic Response Modifiers

Match each definition with its corresponding term. (Note: Not all terms will be used.)

1. _____ Biologic response modifiers that enhance the activity of macrophages and natural killer cells.

2. _____ Cytokines that regulate the growth, differentiation, and function of bone marrow stem cells.

3. _____ Lymphokines, soluble proteins that are released from activated lymphocytes.

4. _____ An immunoglobulin that binds to antigens to form a special complex.

5. _____ A substance that is foreign to the human body.

6. _____ The workhorses of the cellular immune system.

7. _____ The specific cells of the humoral immune system.

a. Colony-stimulating factors

b. Antibody

c. B-cells

d. T-lymphocytes

e. Interferons

f. LAK cells

g. Interleukins

h. Antigen

Choose the *best* answer for each of the following.

8. When are IFN agents usually given?
   a. In the morning, before rising
   b. At mealtimes
   c. Between meals
   d. At bedtime

9. Which agent is used to stimulate the production of red blood cells?
   a. filgrastim
   b. epoetin
   c. sargramostim
   d. interferon beta-1a

10. Which cells are known as the "workhorses" of the cellular immune system?
   a. Plasma cells
   b. B-cells
   c. T-lymphocytes
   d. Memory cells

11. INFs, or interferons, have all the following actions *except*:
   a. antiviral action.
   b. antineoplastic action.
   c. immunomodulation.
   d. immunosuppression.

12. Possible side effects for interferons include all of the following *except*:
   a. sweating.
   b. fever.
   c. chills.
   d. fatigue.

Copyright © 2002 by Mosby, Inc. All rights reserved.

CRITICAL THINKING AND APPLICATION

Answer the following questions on a separate sheet of paper.

13. Ms. Hew is being treated for renal cell carcinoma and is prescribed interleukin-2. Describe an appropriate assessment procedure.

14. Mr. Letti has been receiving the interferon alfa-2b for treatment of Kaposi's sarcoma.

    a. Describe appropriate goals and outcome criteria for Mr. Letti. Do these differ from Ms. Hew's? If so, how? Also, are nursing diagnoses the same for all BRMs?

    b. What—if anything—do you suppose might have been different in Mr. Letti's assessment, as opposed to Ms. Hew's? Were their assessments the same?

15. After a bone marrow transplantation, Mr. Packard is given sargramostim IV. Describe monitoring and other implementation strategies.

Copyright © 2002 by Mosby, Inc. All rights reserved.

Chapter 47

Antacids and Acid Controllers

Match each definition with its corresponding term. (Note: Not all terms will be used.)

1. _____ These agents, known as H$_2$ blockers, reduce stimulated acid secretion.

2. _____ These agents block all acid secretion in the stomach.

3. _____ A cytoprotective agent.

4. _____ The cells are responsible for producing and secreting hydrochloric acid in the stomach.

5. _____ This type of antacid can cause diarrhea.

6. _____ This type of antacid has constipating effects.

7. _____ The cause of many peptic ulcers.

8. _____ Agents used to relieve the painful symptoms associated with gas.

9. _____ This type of antacid may contribute to the development of kidney stones.

10. _____ This agent can result in systemic alkalosis.

a. Aluminum-containing antacids

b. Calcium-containing antacids

c. Magnesium-containing antacids

d. Antiflatulents

e. Proton pump inhibitors

f. *Helicobacter pylori*

g. Sodium bicarbonate

h. Histamine type 2 receptor antagonists

i. Sucralfate

j. Chief cells

k. Parietal cells

Choose the *best* answer for each of the following.

11. Patients who self-medicate with antacids run the risk of:
    a. chronic constipation.
    b. acid-base imbalances due to systemic acidosis.
    c. electrolyte imbalances caused by excessive diarrhea.
    d. masking symptoms of serious underlying diseases, such as bleeding ulcers.

12. Which antacids may be dangerous when taken by patients with renal failure?
    a. Activated charcoal
    b. Aluminum-containing antacids
    c. Calcium-containing antacids
    d. Magnesium-containing antacids

13. Smoking has what effect on patients who are taking medications for ulcer disease?
    a. Smoking has been shown to decrease the effectiveness of H$_2$ blockers.
    b. Smoking has been shown to increase the side effects of H$_2$ blockers.
    c. The actions of antacids are less potent when the patient smokes.
    d. Smoking has no effect on these medications.

Copyright © 2002 by Mosby, Inc. All rights reserved.

14. Which drug would be used as first-line therapy for GERD that has not responded to customary medical treatment?
    a. cimetidine
    b. Mylanta II
    c. omeprazole
    d. sucralfate

15. Which of the following should *not* be included in patient teaching for patients taking omeprazole?
    a. Take the medication before meals.
    b. This medication is intended for long-term therapy.
    c. Take the capsule whole—not crushed, opened, or chewed.
    d. Omeprazole may be given with antacids.

CRITICAL THINKING AND APPLICATION

Answer the following questions on a separate sheet of paper.

16. Mrs. Knopf is advised to take omeprazole to treat her severe case of gastroesophageal reflux disease; nothing else has worked. Develop a patient teaching plan that will inform Mrs. Knopf of potential side/adverse effects. Because she is having so much trouble with her disorder, she is specifically worried about side effects that will further irritate her GI tract.

17. Mr. McKinney has called to ask which antacid he should take. He has been to the store and is confused by the great variety on the shelves. He says he needs something for "occasional heartburn" when he eats something too spicy. He has a history of CHF and is taking antihypertensive drugs. What type of antacid should he take, and what other instructions would he need?

18. Mr. Simmons is taking enteric-coated aspirin for mild arthritis symptoms. He tells you that he plans to take the aspirin with his favorite antacid, Maalox, because he doesn't want any stomach problems. What should you tell him?

Copyright © 2002 by Mosby, Inc. All rights reserved.

Chapter 48

Antidiarrheals and Laxatives

CRITICAL THINKING CROSSWORD

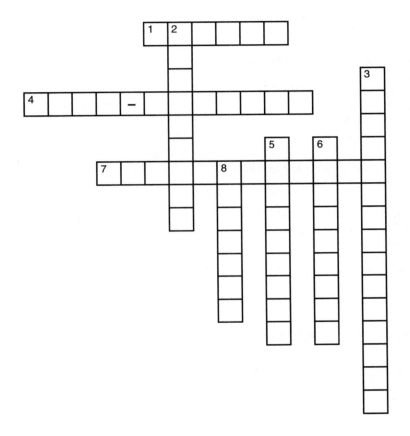

Across

1. Laxatives that increase osmotic pressure in the small intestine, increasing water content and resulting in distension.
4. Laxatives that absorb water into the intestine, increasing bulk and distending the bowel.
7. A laxative that increases fecal water content, resulting in distension, increased peristalsis, and evacuation.

Down

2. Acts by coating the walls of the GI tract, binding to causative bacteria or toxin, and eliminating it via the stool.
3. Acts by decreasing peristalsis and muscular tone of the intestine, thus slowing the movement of substances through the GI tract.
5. A laxative that softens the stool.
6. A laxative that stimulates the nerves that supply the intestine, resulting in increased peristalsis.
8. Also acts to decrease bowel motility.

Copyright © 2002 by Mosby, Inc. All rights reserved.

Choose the *best* answer for each of the following.

1. Which patient should not receive bismuth subsalicylate (Pepto-Bismol)?
   a. Andrew, age 11, who is recovering from the flu
   b. Jeremy, age 22, who has diarrhea after a visit to another country
   c. Joshua, age 43, who complains of constipation
   d. Mark, age 49, who developed diarrhea after a fast-food dinner

2. Which antidiarrheal agent works by decreasing bowel motility?
   a. bismuth subsalicylate (Pepto-Bismol)
   b. loperamide (Imodium)
   c. attapulgite (Kaopectate)
   d. Lactinex

3. Which laxative would be used for the quickest relief of constipation?
   a. Metamucil (psyllium)
   b. Citrucel (methylcellulose)
   c. Colace capsules (docusate sodium)
   d. Senekot (senna)

4. Donald was given PEG-3350 in a solution called GoLytely as preparation for a colonoscopy. He started having diarrhea after about 45 minutes. Two hours later, he calls to tell you that "the diarrhea has not stopped yet." What should you do?
   a. Give him an antidiarrheal agent, such as Lomotil.
   b. Give him another dose of the GoLytely to finish cleansing his bowel.
   c. Remind him that it may take up to 4 hours to completely evacuate the bowel.
   d. Report this to the physician.

5. Bessie, age 79, is visiting the clinic today and tells you that her "bowels just aren't right." She wants advice on the best laxative to take so that she can have a bowel movement every day. Which of the following should you *not* tell her?
   a. A normal bowl pattern does not necessarily mean a bowel movement every day.
   b. Long-term use of laxatives often leads to dependency on laxatives.
   c. If needed, she can take milk of magnesia every day since it is considered mild.
   d. Increasing fluids and fiber in her diet are better alternatives to laxative use.

CRITICAL THINKING AND APPLICATION

Answer the following questions on a separate sheet of paper.

6. Anna has called the health clinic in a panic. She says that she has been taking Pepto-Bismol for diarrhea and noticed this morning that her tongue "is a funny color." She asks, "Have I overdosed on this stuff? What should I do?" What do you tell Anna?

7. Mrs. Benedict is a 65-year-old retiree with osteoporosis and glaucoma. She has recently developed diarrhea, and the physician is considering antidiarrheal therapy. Mrs. Benedict tells you that her husband recently "had a bout with diarrhea" for which he took Donnatal. Mrs. Benedict wonders whether Donnatal would help in her case. What do you tell her?

8. Charles recently completed a round of antibiotic therapy and now has diarrhea that the physician suspects was caused by the antibiotic.

   a. What antidiarrheal agent is indicated for Charles?

   b. Does he also need a different antibiotic to eliminate the *Lactobacillus* in his GI tract?

9. Hillary has come to the physician's office complaining of constipation. During your assessment, Hillary mentions that she recently started graduate school and hasn't had time lately to keep up her usual exercise regimen—and her diet is a "disaster." She says that, on some days, all she has time to do is grab a milkshake at the student union. She also tells you that she has been taking antacids for "heartburn." What might be causing Hillary's constipation?

Copyright © 2002 by Mosby, Inc. All rights reserved.

10. Ira, a 45-year-old accountant, has chronic constipation.

    a. What are the advantages of the bulk-forming laxatives in treating Ira?

    b. The physician prescribes psyllium. What instructions do you give Ira regarding its administration?

11. Drake is a 5-year-old boy with constipation. The physician has ordered treatment with glycerin suppositories.

    a. Why is glycerin a good choice for Drake?

    b. What adverse effects will you monitor for?

12. Five-year-old Kyle has diarrhea for which the physician has ordered an antidiarrheal agent.

    a. How will the dosage likely be determined?

    b. The next day Kyle's mother calls to tell you that Kyle seems to be no better and that his abdomen "looks bloated" and is painful. What do you do?

Copyright © 2002 by Mosby, Inc. All rights reserved.

Chapter 49

Antiemetic (Antinausea) Agents

Choose the *best* answer for each of the following.

1. Which agents may also cause drowsiness and drying of secretions when given to reduce nausea?
   a. Antihistamines
   b. Neuroleptics
   c. Serotonin blockers
   d. THC

2. Which class of antinausea agents has proven to be very effective in preventing chemotherapy-induced nausea and vomiting?
   a. Antihistamines
   b. Neuroleptics
   c. Serotonin blockers
   d. THC

3. Which agent is a synthetic derivative of the major active substance in marijuana?
   a. ondansetron
   b. metoclopramide
   c. prochlorperazine
   d. dronabinol

4. Antiemetics that are used to prevent nausea and vomiting in patients undergoing chemotherapy are most effective when given:
   a. before meals.
   b. at bedtime.
   c. before the chemotherapy begins.
   d. just after the chemotherapy begins.

5. Patients taking dronabinol should be reminded to be aware of which possible side effect?
   a. Palpitations
   b. Orthostatic hypotension
   c. Diarrhea
   d. Difficult urination

CRITICAL THINKING AND APPLICATION

Answer the following questions on a separate sheet of paper.

6. Norman, who has Parkinson's disease, is experiencing nausea and vomiting. Why might a neuroleptic agent not be a good choice for Norman?

7. Petra has gastroesophageal reflux, and the physician has ordered oral metoclopramide.

   a. What instructions do you give Petra for administration of the medication?

   b. A few days later, Petra calls to say that she thinks the medication is "too strong." She also mentions that her evening routine includes "a couple of glasses of wine." What do you tell Petra?

8. Mr. Ontkin has been prescribed ondansetron during his chemotherapy.

   a. What significant drug interactions should you assess for?

   b. One day Mr. Ontkin complains to you that he gets a headache every time the ondansetron is administered. What should you do?

Copyright © 2002 by Mosby, Inc. All rights reserved.

9. Nellie, a patient on your unit, has been prescribed thiethylperazine maleate. You are preparing the injection when Nellie says, "I hate shots. Can't you just add that to my IV?" What is your response, and how will you administer the agent?

Chapter 50

Vitamins and Minerals

Match each definition with its corresponding term.

1. _____ Specialized protein that catalyzes chemical reactions in organic matter.

2. _____ A deficiency of cyanocobalamin.

3. _____ A nonprotein substance that combines with a protein molecule to form an active enzyme.

4. _____ A condition caused by a vitamin D deficiency that is characterized by soft, pliable bones.

5. _____ An inorganic substance ingested and attached to enzymes or other organic molecules.

6. _____ An organic compound essential in small quantities for normal physiologic and metabolic functioning in the body.

7. _____ A condition resulting from an ascorbic acid deficiency that is characterized by weakness and anemia.

8. _____ An essential organic compound that can be dissolved and stored in the liver and fatty tissues.

9. _____ A biologically active chemical that combines with others to make up vitamin E compounds.

10. _____ A disease of the peripheral nerves caused by an inability to assimilate thiamine.

11. _____ An essential organic compound that can be dissolved in water but is not stored in the body for long periods of time.

12. _____ A disease resulting from a niacin or tryptophan deficiency or a metabolic defect that interferes with conversion of tryptophan to niacin.

a. Beriberi

b. Coenzyme

c. Enzyme

d. Fat-soluble vitamin

e. Mineral

f. Pellagra

g. Pernicious anemia

h. Rickets

i. Scurvy

j. Tocopherol

k. Vitamin

l. Water-soluble vitamin

Choose the *best* answer for each of the following.

13. Which vitamin can become toxic if consumed in excess amounts?
    a. vitamin A
    b. vitamin C
    c. niacin
    d. folic acid

Copyright © 2002 by Mosby, Inc. All rights reserved.

14. Cindi believes that taking megadoses of vitamin C is healthy. She should be aware that megadoses:
    a. are usually nontoxic because vitamin C is water-soluble.
    b. can produce nausea, vomiting, headache, and abdominal cramps.
    c. can lead to scurvy-like symptoms.
    d. may cause dangerous heart dysrhythmias.

15. If excessive amounts of water-soluble vitamins are ingested, what usually happens?
    a. The body will store them in muscle and fat tissue until needed.
    b. They are stored in the liver until needed.
    c. They circulate in the blood, bound to proteins, until needed.
    d. Excess amounts are excreted in the urine.

16. Symptoms of magnesium deficiency include all the following *except*:
    a. cardiovascular disturbances.
    b. neuromuscular impairment.
    c. renal insufficiency.
    d. mental impairment.

17. The efficient absorption of calcium in the diet requires adequate amounts of:
    a. phosphorus.
    b. intrinsic factor.
    c. coenzymes.
    d. vitamin D.

CRITICAL THINKING AND APPLICATION

Answer the following questions on a separate sheet of paper.

18. Mrs. Steinman has developed vitamin D deficiency as the result of long-term use of lubricant laxatives. She is advised to take supplements for her vitamin D deficiency. However, the physician also advises her to get vitamin D through more natural sources, both dietary and endogenous. "What did he mean by 'endogenous'?" she asks you. Explain to Mrs. Steinman what is meant by an endogenous source, and make her a list of foods rich in vitamin D as well.

19. After Mr. Wang's treatment with a broad-spectrum antibiotic, he begins to show signs of vitamin K deficiency.

    a. Why?

    b. What function does vitamin K serve in the human body?

    c. Despite its infrequent occurrences, what other patient populations can sometimes be at risk for this deficiency?

    d. Finally, what dietary supplements can you recommend?

20. Ms. Evans has recently had an ileal resection, which is, understandably, affecting her digestive functions. She is experiencing some small signs of malabsorption. When you run routine laboratory tests you discover that she is mildly anemic. What do you expect? Create a hand-held patient education card for Ms. Evans, concentrating on diet. Be sure to include a list of foods that contain the vitamin or vitamins from which she is most likely to suffer a deficiency.

21. Mr. Graham is hospitalized with severe hypocalcemia. Your colleague Jeffrey recommends an immediate start of rapidly infused IV calcium. The physician's order requires infusion with 1% procaine. Refute or defend the rationale of both Jeffrey and Mr. Graham's physician. In either case, what should you watch out for when giving IV calcium? Back up your response with your own data.

Copyright © 2002 by Mosby, Inc. All rights reserved.

Chapter 51

Nutritional Supplements

CRITICAL THINKING CROSSWORD

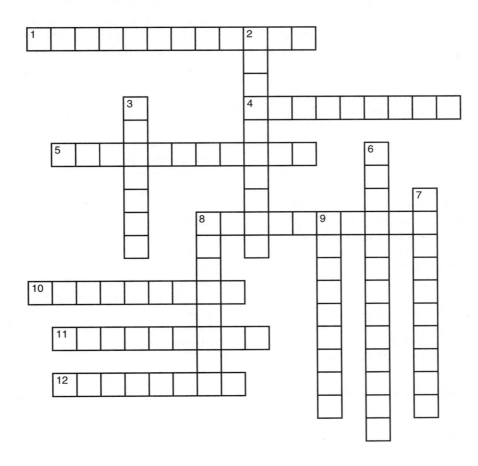

Across

1. Mr. George is receiving _____ when it is determined that he is going to need nutritional supplementation as well. When you see that he is taking this drug, however, you ask if feeding can wait till his other drug therapy has run its course, because the nutritional supplement will inactivate this drug because of high gastric acid content or prolonged emptying time.

4. Ms. Carter needs amino acids in nutritional supplements. The main use, or primary role, of amino acids is _____.

5. Mr. Harris is about to receive a _____, in which a feeding tube will be surgically inserted directly into his stomach.

8. Mrs. Page is worried about her husband with post-surgical nausea. She sees that his roommate is receiving TPN and asks "Can't you do that for my husband just while he's so nauseated?" TPN, you explain, is to be used only when enteral support is impossible or when the GI tract's _____ or functional capacity is insufficient.

10. Ms. Cedaras comes to the clinic when a cut on her hand "just won't heal up." She also says that as long as she's here, she'd like to report symptoms of hair loss and scaly dermatitis. She wants a prescription for her skin problem, but the physician says, "There's something more going on here." He runs a few tests and discovers that Ms. Cedaras also has decreased

Copyright © 2002 by Mosby, Inc. All rights reserved.

platelets and some evidence of possible fatty liver. He says he suspects Ms. Cedaras has essential _____ deficiency *(two words)*.

11. Mr. Hill is having trouble getting and digesting enough dietary forms of amino acids. His physician explains that he needs nutritional supplementation through enteral nutrition to ensure that he gets enough of these amino acids, since they cannot be produced by his own body. Mr. Hill is suffering from a deficiency of _____ amino acids.

12. Craig, a college sophomore, takes a great deal of interest in the supplementary nutrition he is receiving and asks to read the label. He says, "There are some amino acids missing from this. Why aren't you giving me all of them?" You explain that some amino acids, all but eight, in fact, are manufactured in the body, using _____ sources.

Down

2. When Ms. Carter asks why she needs amino acid supplemental feedings, you explain that amino acids promote growth and help with wound healing. One of the principle ways they do so is by reducing or slowing the breakdown of proteins, or _____.

3. The Johnsons recently appeared in a TV commercial because they drink Ensure to take care of a few extra nutritional needs they have experienced with aging. Their nephew recently had surgery; while recovering, he received a nasogastric delivery of a modular formulation to supplement a polymeric feeding formulation he needed. When their grandson was an infant, his parents supplemented his breastfeeding with an infant nutritional formulation. Each member of the Johnson clan discussed here has received some form of _____ nutrition.

6. What type of amino acid is Lauren from 8 Down receiving?

7. You are explaining to Mrs. Glendale's family that the parenteral nutritional supplementation you are about to institute will help her by bypassing the entire GI system, eliminating the need for absorption and _____.

8. Lauren, age 10, is going through a period of rapid growth. She is receiving enough essential amino acids in her diet, and her body has no problems producing its normal levels of nonessential amino acids. Nevertheless, she is to receive an amino acid that is not produced in large enough quantities to support this rapid growth spurt. Lauren is to receive a supplemental source of _____.

9. Mr. Kennedy has been receiving peripheral parenteral nutrition. One day something rather rare occurs: his vein becomes inflamed. You notify the physician. "Left untreated," she tells you, "this could have become really severe. He could even have lost his arm eventually, if you hadn't caught this so quickly." Mr. Kennedy, of course, has _____.

Choose the *best* answer for each of the following.

1. The maximum percentage of dextrose in peripheral TPN infusions should be:
   a. 10%.
   b. 20%.
   c. 50%.
   d. 100%.

2. Ensure and Sustacal are examples of:
   a. elemental or monomeric solutions.
   b. blenderized solutions.
   c. polymeric, lactose-free solutions.
   d. polymeric, milk-based solutions.

3. All of the following are potential complications of TPN *except*:
   a. pneumothorax.
   b. aspiration.
   c. hyperglycemia.
   d. infection.

4. The most common side effect and adverse effect of enteral nutritional supplements is:
   a. anorexia.
   b. constipation.
   c. diarrhea.
   d. flatulence.

5. Which of the following is an indication for peripheral TPN?
   a. Short-term delivery of TPN (less than 2 weeks)
   b. Long-term delivery of TPN (more than 2 weeks)
   c. Patients with severe nutritional problems
   d. Patients who wish to reduce their weight

Copyright © 2002 by Mosby, Inc. All rights reserved.

6. Which statement about enteral feedings is true?
   a. Check gastric residual volumes once a day.
   b. Begin the infusions at the maximum rate ordered.
   c. The head of the bed should remain flat.
   d. Tube feeding formulas should be at room temperature.

CRITICAL THINKING AND APPLICATION

Answer the following questions on a separate sheet of paper.

7. Ms. Schiller has one of the newer tubes for nasogastric feeding.

   a. What are the advantages and disadvantages of these newer tubes?

   b. The first time you try to perform a gastric aspiration on Ms. Schiller, you are unsuccessful. What should you do?

8. Mr. Robbins, who is on TPN therapy, manifests a weak pulse, hypertension, tachycardia, and decreased urine output. He seems somewhat confused, and you note, on examining him, that he exhibits pitting edema. What's wrong? Can you do anything about it? What could you have done differently to avoid this reaction?

Copyright © 2002 by Mosby, Inc. All rights reserved.

Chapter 52

Blood-Forming Agents

Choose the *best* answer for each of the following.

1. Intrinsic RBC abnormalities, which lead to anemias, may be due to:
   a. G6PD deficiency.
   b. DIC.
   c. use of intraaortic balloon pumps.
   d. drug-induced antibodies.

2. Patients who take iron preparations should be warned of the possible side effects, which may include:
   a. dizziness and orthostatic hypotension.
   b. nausea, vomiting, diarrhea, and stomach cramps.
   c. drowsiness, lethargy, and fatigue.
   d. neuropathy and tingling in the extremities.

3. What happens if folic acid is given to treat anemias without determining the underlying cause of the anemia?
   a. Erythropoiesis is inhibited.
   b. Excessive levels of folic acid may accumulate, causing toxicity.
   c. The symptoms of pernicious anemia may be masked, delaying treatment.
   d. Intrinsic factor is destroyed.

4. Indications for folic acid include all the following *except*:
   a. megaloblastic anemia.
   b. tropical sprue.
   c. prophylaxis of fetal neural tube defects.
   d. pernicious anemia.

5. Which of the following would *not* be included in the teaching for patients who take oral iron preparations?
   a. Mix the liquid iron preparations with antacids to reduce GI distress.
   b. Take the iron with meals if GI distress occurs.
   c. Liquid forms should be taken with a straw to avoid discoloration of tooth enamel.
   d. Oral forms should be taken with juice, not milk.

CRITICAL THINKING AND APPLICATION

Answer the following questions on a separate sheet of paper.

6. Mr. Dlugy is prescribed iron dextran IM. However, before you can give him his first injection, the pharmacist suggests you give him a smaller dose of 25 mg first. Why does she suggest this? How should IM iron dextran be administered?

7. You are aware of the foods that contain iron. What other foods may either enhance the intake of iron, or perhaps hinder it?

8. Four-year-old David has accidentally ingested an oral iron preparation. Describe the treatment plan. What if the serum iron concentration is >300 µg/dl? Does that affect the treatment plan?

9. Describe the treatment for a child with more severe symptoms of iron intoxication than those seen in David (question 8). In this case, please first describe the most severe intoxication symptoms and then the treatment response.

135

Copyright © 2002 by Mosby, Inc. All rights reserved.

Chapter 53

Dermatologic Agents

Choose the *best* answer for each of the following.

1. Which of the following statements accurately describes antifungal therapy for topical infections?
   a. Treatment may be needed for several weeks to as long as a year to eradicate the organism.
   b. Antifungal therapy works best when the affected area is exposed to sunlight.
   c. Oral agents are the preferred agents for treating topical fungal infections.
   d. Antifungal therapy is palliative only; fungi are rarely eradicated from topical areas.

2. Miconazole suppositories for vaginal yeast infections should be used as follows:
   a. 200-mg suppositories inserted every other day at bedtime.
   b. 200-mg suppositories inserted once daily at bedtime for 3 consecutive days.
   c. a one-time dose of 200 mg administered in the morning.
   d. 100-mg suppositories inserted every night at bedtime until symptoms stop.

3. Ms. Lauder, who has a rash, needs a medication that will cover a large area of her body; however, her skin is tender to the touch. If each has the same healing properties, which of the following formulations might be preferred for Ms. Lauder?
   a. Aerosol spray
   b. Gel
   c. Oil
   d. Tape

4. Ms. Thierry needs a medication that has excellent emollient properties. Because she works as a swimming coach, the medication prescribed should not wash off when it comes in contact with water. If each has the same healing properties, which of the following formulations would be preferred for Ms. Thierry?
   a. Tape
   b. Oil
   c. Gel
   d. Lotion

5. Which of the following statements about topical antiviral agents is *not* true?
   a. Common side effects include stinging, itching, and rash.
   b. Topically applied acyclovir does not cure viral skin infections but does seem to decrease the healing time and pain.
   c. Topically applied acyclovir can cure viral skin infections if applied as soon as symptoms appear.
   d. They are applied topically for the treatment of both initial and recurrent herpes simplex infections.

137

Copyright © 2002 by Mosby, Inc. All rights reserved.

CRITICAL THINKING AND APPLICATION

Answer the following questions on a separate sheet of paper.

6. Mr. Mugler has a topical skin infection. He is prescribed clindamycin. He has never used this drug before. You realize that it's a good idea to assess him for possible sensitivity or allergies. What precautions can you take?

7. You are getting ready to apply erythromycin to a patient's skin. The affected area of the skin is not oozing or even moist, but your supervisor still requires that you wear gloves. Why?

8. Ms. Goodman is to receive methylprednisolone to treat an inflammation of the skin. You will be using occlusive dressings as part of her treatment. Describe the appropriate implementation strategies.

9. Mr. Lacroix's two children have brought "something" home from school, and by the time he brings them into the clinic, he has "it" too! He tells you he has used lindane on everyone's scalps, but he has come in because he wants his children and himself checked, because he is not confident that he has "taken care of things properly." What are Mr. Lacroix and his children being treated for? Describe for him basic steps in using this product. What other measures should he take?

10. With a partner, develop two different case studies of acne patients. Assign one patient benzoyl peroxide, the other tretinoin. What differences in implementation and precautions do you come up with as a result?

Copyright © 2002 by Mosby, Inc. All rights reserved.

Chapter 54

Ophthalmic Agents

Match each definition with its corresponding term. (Note: Not all terms will be used.)

1. _____ Adjustment of the eye to variation in distance.

2. _____ Inflammation of the eyelids.

3. _____ The clear, watery fluid that circulates in the anterior and posterior chambers of the eye.

4. _____ An abnormal condition of the lens of the eye, characterized by loss of transparency.

5. _____ Paralysis of the ciliary muscles, which prevents accommodation of the lens to variations in distance.

6. _____ Excessive intraocular pressure caused by elevated levels of aqueous humor.

7. _____ The mucous membrane that lines the eyelids.

8. _____ Drugs that constrict the pupil.

9. _____ Iris, ciliary body, and choroids of the eye.

10. _____ Drugs that dilate the pupil.

a. Cycloplegia

b. Conjunctiva

c. Accommodation

d. Glaucoma

e. Mydriatics

f. Miotics

g. Uvea

h. Blepharitis

i. Vitreous humor

j. Aqueous humor

k. Cataract

Choose the _best_ answer for each of the following.

11. Which ophthalmic agents are contraindicated if the patient is allergic to sulfa drugs?
    a. Beta blockers
    b. Osmotic diuretics
    c. Carbonic anhydrase inhibitors
    d. Prostaglandins

12. What is the purpose of acetylcholine?
    a. Produces mydriasis for ophthalmic examinations
    b. Produces immediate miosis during ophthalmic surgery
    c. Causes cycloplegia to allow for measurement of IOP
    d. Acts as a topical anesthetic during ophthalmic surgery

13. Patients taking latanoprost should be advised of which of the following possible side effects?
    a. Temporary eye color changes, from light eye colors to brown
    b. Permanent eye color changes, from light eye colors to brown
    c. Photosensitivity
    d. Bradycardia and hypotension

14. Willis has come to the emergency room with an eye injury. After the application of fluorescein, the physician sees an area with a green halo. What does this indicate?
    a. A corneal defect
    b. A conjunctival lesion
    c. The presence of a hard contact lens
    d. A foreign object

139

Copyright © 2002 by Mosby, Inc. All rights reserved.

15. Which of the following is *not* true regarding application of ophthalmic preparations?
    a. Apply drops directly to the cornea.
    b. Apply drops into the conjunctival sac.
    c. Apply pressure to the inner canthus for 1 minute after medication administration.
    d. Apply ointments in a thin layer.

CRITICAL THINKING AND APPLICATION

Answer the following questions on a separate sheet of paper.

16. Jonathan has blue eyes; Julie has brown eyes. Why would the drug effects of the miotics on the iris be less pronounced in Julie?

17. The physician is planning long-term echothiophate therapy for Patrice.

    a. What patient teaching is important in this situation?

    b. Several months later, Patrice comes to the ER with difficulty breathing, bradycardia, and hypotension. She also says that she "can't see!" Is it possible that Patrice is exhibiting toxic effects from her topical ophthalmic medication? Explain your answer.

    c. What treatment is indicated for Patrice in the event of toxicity involving a miotic?

18. Mrs. Ngo, a 60-year-old librarian, has open-angle glaucoma. The physician prescribes Propine.

    a. Why might the physician have chosen that agent over epinephrine?

    b. What problems will you tell Mrs. Ngo to report?

    c. Do you expect any serious reactions to the drug? Explain your answer.

19. The physician prescribes a beta-adrenergic blocker for Ned, who has ocular hypertension. Ned has what he calls "an allergic reaction" to the drug, and the physician changes his medication to another beta-blocking drug, timolol. Since both of these agents are beta-adrenergic blockers, and Ned had a reaction to the first agent, why would the physician merely switch Ned to another drug in the same category?

20. Mrs. O'Rourke, who has acute narrow-angle glaucoma, has been scheduled for an iridectomy.

    a. What agent is indicated, and how is it administered?

    b. Following administration of the agent, you find Mrs. O'Rourke sitting up in bed, complaining of a headache. How could her headache be diminished?

21. You are preparing to administer sulfacetamide to Tony, a patient with an eye infection.

    a. Why will you cleanse Tony's eye before administering the medication?

    b. Before using the sulfacetamide, you examine it, then throw the solution away and look for another container of sulfacetamide. Why did you do that?

22. Louisa has an inflammatory disorder of the eye for which the physician has prescribed a topical nonsteroidal antiinflammatory ophthalmic agent. Why might the physician have chosen an NSAID over a corticosteroid?

23. Ms. Luna has been prescribed ophthalmic corticosteroid drops for an inflammation of her eye. The next day she calls the clinic and tells you, "These drops sting so much when I use them that I can't even put my contacts in." What is your advice?

Copyright © 2002 by Mosby, Inc. All rights reserved.

Chapter 55

Otic Agents

Choose the *best* answer for each of the following.

1. Common symptoms of otitis media include all the following *except*:
   a. pain.
   b. fever.
   c. ear drainage.
   d. hearing loss.

2. Middle ear infections generally require treatment with:
   a. topical steroids.
   b. systemic steroids.
   c. topical antibiotics.
   d. systemic antibiotics.

3. Preparations that soften and help eliminate cerumen are known as:
   a. antifungals.
   b. wax emulsifiers.
   c. steroids.
   d. local analgesics.

4. Contraindications to otic preparations, such as chloramphenicol, include:
   a. eardrum perforation.
   b. the presence of *Pseudomonas aeruginosa*.
   c. the presence of *Staphylococcus aureus*.
   d. mastoiditis.

5. In children, what usually precedes episodes of otitis media?
   a. Water sports
   b. Foreign objects
   c. Upper respiratory tract infection
   d. Mastoiditis

CRITICAL THINKING AND APPLICATION

Answer the following questions on a separate sheet of paper.

6. A patient calls the physician's office complaining of severe pain in and drainage from his left ear. He also says he "had a little mishap" on his motorcycle yesterday. What do you tell him?

7. Why are antiinfective agents frequently combined with steroids?

8. Andre, a 30-year-old teacher, has an ear infection for which chloramphenicol has been prescribed.

   a. What do you do before you instill the drops?

   b. If Andre were 10 years old rather than 30, how would the dosage be adjusted?

   c. What do you warn Andre might happen after the drops are instilled?

9. Mrs. Franz, a 52-year-old office manager, has come to the clinic today complaining of a painful, "itchy" left ear. The physician diagnoses an infection of the external auditory canal and prescribes a topical antibiotic.

   a. What is the advantage of using a product containing hydrocortisone?

   b. What would be a contraindication to Mrs. Franz's use of this type of agent?

141

Copyright © 2002 by Mosby, Inc. All rights reserved.

10. Why do so many otic combination products contain local anesthetic agents?

11. Ben is a 3-year-old preschooler, and his brother Drew is a 6-year-old kindergartner. They both require otic agents for ear infections.

    a. What instructions do you give the boys' parents regarding instillation of the drops?

    b. A few days later, the boys' mother brings them back for a follow-up visit. Ben and Drew don't seem to be in pain, and there is no redness or swelling in either child's ears. What does this mean?

12. During a home visit, you observe Esther's husband preparing her eardrops. He puts a glass of water in the microwave, telling you that he will soak the bottle of eardrops in hot water to warm them up.

    a. How is Esther's husband doing so far?

    b. Later, right after her husband instills the drops, Esther sits up and asks you whether they are now doing everything right. What do you tell her?

Copyright © 2002 by Mosby, Inc. All rights reserved.

Overview of Dosage Calculations

There are many important aspects to consider when doing calculations, but probably the most important one is common sense. If a drug dose calculation does not seem right, then most likely it is not. The administration of drugs to patients is a shared responsibility among the patient, physician, pharmacist, and nurse. All those involved have a moral and legal responsibility to ensure that the administration takes place in a safe and effective way. The nurse has a legal and a professional responsibility to ensure that his or her patients receive the right dose of the right medication at the right time and in the right manner. There are many checks and balances in the system to guarantee that this happens. The necessary basic calculations involved in the safe and accurate administration of medications to patients are described in this section.

Calculating drug doses is one small part of the overall process of pharmacologic therapy. Before you actually calculate a drug dose, you must follow many steps. The nurse should evaluate the patient and the prescribed medication for the five "rights": right patient, right drug, right dose, right time, and right route. Other principles to follow to decrease the likelihood of mistakes are to calculate doses systematically and to do your calculations consistently time after time so that the process becomes easier with each calculation. It also helps to have a peer check your calculations, especially if the dose seems unusual or if the math is very difficult. Remember, common sense should prevail. If a calculation shows that you should give 25 mg of digoxin and the strongest strength is 0.25 mg, common sense should tell you that the patient should not be given 100 pills, especially since drug dosage forms are usually manufactured with the most commonly prescribed dosages in mind.

You must have basic arithmetic skills before beginning. The following basic principles may need to be reviewed:

➢ Basic multiplication
➢ Basic division
➢ Roman numerals
➢ Fractions (reducing to lowest terms, addition, subtraction, multiplication, division, mixed numbers)
➢ Decimals (adding, subtracting, multiplication, division)
➢ Ratios and percentages (changing a fraction to a percentage, changing a ratio to a percentage)
➢ Solving for "x" in a simple equation

RULES TO REMEMBER

❖ Before calculating a drug dose for a particular patient, you must first convert all units of measure to a SINGLE system, if this has not already been done. For example, do NOT attempt to guess which is correct if the drug is ordered in grains but the drug label is in milligrams. The best approach is to convert to the system used on the drug label. You may have to convert the patient's weight from pounds to kilograms if the medication is ordered to be given per kilogram of weight.

❖ **Rounding.** Always round your answers to the nearest dose that is *measurable*, after verifying that the dose is correct for that patient.

• If a tablet is scored, you may round to the nearest half tablet.
Example: 1.8 tablets, give 2 tablets
1.2 tablets, give 1 tablet

• If a tablet is unscored, call the pharmacy. Recheck your calculations if the dose is more than 1 or 2 tablets. It is very difficult, if not impossible, to cut an unscored tablet into fourths accurately.

• To round liquids, *look at the equipment you plan to use.* Some syringes are marked in tenths or hundredths of a milliliter. Larger syringes are marked in 0.2-ml increments. Tuberculin syringes are marked in hundredths. For liquid medications, NEVER round up to the nearest WHOLE number. If the answer is 1.8 ml, DO NOT round up to 2 ml. Rounding up in these situations may lead to overdosing. However, if you are using an electronic infusion pump, you will probably need to round to the nearest whole number.

143

Copyright © 2002 by Mosby, Inc. All rights reserved.

- To round to the nearest tenth, look at the hundredths column. If it is 0.5 or more, round UP to the next tenth.
  Example: To round to the nearest tenth:
  1.78 or 1.75, round to 1.8
  1.32 or 1.34, round to 1.3
- A syringe calibrated in hundredths permits more exact measurement of small dosages. To round to the nearest hundredth, look at the thousandth column. If it is 0.005 or more, round UP to the next hundredth.
  Example: To round to the nearest hundredth:
  1.847, round to 1.85
  1.653, round to 1.65
- NOTE: Never round up liquid medications to the nearest whole number. If the answer is 1.6 ml, DO NOT round up to 2 ml! Such increases may lead to overdoses.
- PEDIATRIC DOSES are rounded to the TENTHS place, not whole numbers. Rounding to whole numbers may lead to overdoses.

❖ **Leading Zeros.** Always insert a zero (0) in front of decimals when the number is less than a whole number. This draws attention to the decimal and avoids potential errors.
  Example: 0.05 is CORRECT.
  .05 is NOT correct.

❖ **Labeling.** Always label your answers with the appropriate unit. If the problems asked for a number of tablets, write "tablets." If you are to give an injection, use "ml" or "cc." Heparin and insulin, however, use "units" instead of "mg" or "μg." Intravenous drips will either be written in terms of "ml/hr" or "gtt/cc." Problems using an intravenous infusion pump are ALWAYS asking for ml/hr. THINK about what the question is asking, and then label your answer appropriately.

❖ **Common Sense.** Use common sense! Drug companies typically formulate medications that are close to the usual doses and medications that can provide the ordered dose with one or two tablets. If your answer indicates that you should give 60 ml IM, CHECK IT AGAIN! Remember, you can only give 2 to 3 ml IM, depending on institution policies, so a dosage of 60 ml would be inappropriate.

INTERPRETING MEDICATION LABELS

Medication labels contain a great amount of information—much of it in small print. The drug manufacturer prints some labels; others are prepared by pharmacy technicians or pharmacists for institutional use. The most important information is as follows:

- Generic name—the first letter is usually lower-cased. This is the name used by all companies that produce the drug.
- Trade, brand, or proprietary name—the first letter is usually capitalized. This name is used only by the manufacturer of the drug and may be followed by the "®" symbol.
- Unit dose per milliliter, per tablet, per capsule, etc.
- Total amount in the container
- Route
- Directions for preparation, if needed
- Directions for storage
- Expiration date

Other information, such as a specification for adult or pediatric use, may be noted on the label.

Copyright © 2002 by Mosby, Inc. All rights reserved.

Example:

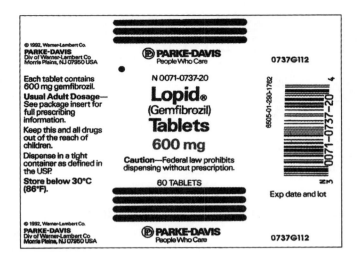

Generic name:	gemfibrozil
Trade name:	Lopid
Unit dose:	600 mg per tablet
Total amount in container:	60 tablets
Route:	(It is assumed that tablets are oral route.)

For the following labels, identify the information requested:

1.

NDC 0068-0508-30

300 mg | MARION MERRELL DOW INC.

RIFADIN®
(rifampin capsules)

300 mg

30 Capsules

Each capsule contains: rifampin..............................300 mg
Usual Dose: See accompanying product information.
CAUTION: Federal law prohibits dispensing without prescription.
Keep tightly closed. Store in a dry place. Avoid excessive heat.
Dispense in tight, light-resistant container with child-resistant closure.

© 1993 Marion Merrell Dow Inc.

Merrell Dow Pharmaceuticals Inc.
Subsidiary of Marion Merrell Dow Inc.
Kansas City, MO 64114   H 3 6 4 C

Generic name:	_____
Trade name:	_____
Unit dose:	_____
Total amount in container:	_____
Route:	_____

2.

NDC 0002-5136-18
75 mL (When Mixed)   M-5136

℞ *Lilly*

LORABID®
LORACARBEF
FOR ORAL
SUSPENSION, USP

200 mg
per 5 mL

CAUTION—Federal (USA)
law prohibits dispensing
without prescription.

Generic name:	_____
Trade name:	_____
Unit dose:	_____
Total amount in container:	_____
Route:	_____

Copyright © 2002 by Mosby, Inc. All rights reserved.

3.

> For IM use only
> See package insert for complete product information
> Shake vigorously immediately before each use
> 812 224 302
>
> The Upjohn Company
> Kalamazoo, MI 49001 USA
>
> Upjohn   NDC 0009-0626-01
> 2.5 mL Vial
> **Depo-Provera®**
> Sterile Aqueous Suspension
> sterile medroxyprogesterone
> acetate suspension, USP
>
> **400mg per mL**

Generic name: _____

Trade name: _____

Unit dose: _____

Total amount in container: _____

Route: _____

SECTION I: BASIC CONVERSIONS USING RATIO AND PROPORTION

A proportion is a way of stating a relationship of equality between two ratios. The first ratio listed is EQUAL to the second ratio listed. The double colon (::) that separates the two ratios means AS. The numbers at each end of the ratio equation can be called the "outside," and the two numbers in the middle of the ratio (around the "::") can be called the "inside." Ratio and proportion problems can be used to calculate ONE of the numbers in the equation if it is not known. The simple rule to use is this:

The product of the outside terms equals the product of the inside terms.

If one of the terms is not known, it is designated as "*x*." The problem is then set up to solve for "*x*."

Example:

1 : 100 :: 4 : *x*   means:

"The relationship of 1 to 100 is the same as the relationship of 4 to *x*." The "*x*" is unknown.

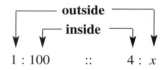

1 and *x* are the "outsides;" 100 and 4 are the "insides." To solve for "*x*," multiply the "outsides" (1 × *x*) together, multiply the "insides" (100 × 4) together, and form an equation:

$(1 \times x) = (100 \times 4)$

$1x = 400$

$x = 400$

Proof: You may prove your equation as follows: Insert the answer for "*x*" in the original equation, then solve.

1 × 400 = 400 (outsides)

100 × 4 = 400 (insides)

400 = 400; the answer for "*x*" is correct.

Copyright © 2002 by Mosby, Inc. All rights reserved.

Example:

5 : 25 :: 15 : x
Multiply the "outsides" and the "insides" and form an equation; then solve for x.
$(5 \times x) = (25 \times 15)$
$5x = 375$
$x = 375/5$
$x = 75$

Proof:

$5 \times 75 = 375$
$25 \times 15 = 375$
$375 = 375$

Calculating ratios is one of the major foundations of drug dosage calculations. When calculating a dosage, the nurse will use the medication on hand to calculate how much of it to give for a desired dosage. The nurse uses the principle of proportion to accurately calculate how much medication to give. The following chart provides a few common equivalents used in pharmacology. These equivalents are then used in ratio and proportion problems to calculate appropriate dosages.

BASIC EQUIVALENTS

Metric Equivalents	Approximate Equivalents
Weight 1 mg = 1000 µg or mcg (micrograms) 1 g = 1000 mg (milligrams) 1 kg = 1000 g (grams)	1 gr (grain) = 60 mg 1000 mg = 1 g = gr xv (15)
Volume 1000 ml (or cc) = 1 L	1 tsp = 5 ml 1 tbsp = 15 ml 2 tbsp = 30 ml 1 oz = 30 ml 1 kg = 2.2 lb 1 cc = 1 ml (weighs approximately 1 g)

To find basic equivalents from one unit of measure to another, use the ratio and proportion approach.

Example 1: The drug dosage is 500 mg. You have scored tablets on hand that are 1 g each. How many tablets will you give?

You have *grams* on hand. You need to change the *milligrams* needed to the equivalent *grams* on hand. Find the proper equivalents:
     Equivalent: 1 g = 1000 mg
Next, set up the ratio and proportion equation.
     On the LEFT side put the ratio that you ***know***: 1 g is 1000 mg
     On the RIGHT side, put the ratio that you ***want to know***: how many g ("x") is 500 mg?
Know   ***Want to Know***
1 g : 1000 mg :: x g : 500 mg
Solve for x: $(1 \times 500) = (1000 \times x)$; $500 = 1000x$; $x = 500/1000$; $x = 0.5$
You will give 0.5 (half) of the 1-g tablet.
To double-check your answer, substitute your answer for the x and solve. The "outsides" should equal the "insides."
     $1 \times 500 = 500$; $1000 \times 0.5 = 500$; $500 = 500$

Copyright © 2002 by Mosby, Inc. All rights reserved.

Example 2: Cough syrup, 45 ml, is ordered. The cough syrup comes in a 2-oz bottle. How many ounces do you give?

> You have ounces on hand. You need to give 45 ml.
> Equivalent: 1 oz = 30 ml
> **Know:** 1 oz is 30 ml; **Want to Know**: How many ounces is 45 ml?
> **Know**   **Want to Know**
> 1 oz : 30 ml :: x oz : 45 ml
> $(1 \times 45) = (30 \times x)$; $45 = 30x$; $x = 45/30 = 1.5$ oz = 45 ml
> **Proof:** $1 \times 45 = 45$; $30 \times 1.5 = 45$; $45 = 45$

Example 3: Mabel weighs 122 lb. How many kilograms does she weigh?

> Equivalent: 1 kg = 2.2 lb
> **Know**   **Want to Know**
> 1 kg : 2.2 lb :: x kg : 122 lb
> $(1 \times 122) = (2.2 \times x)$; $122 = 2.2x$; $122/2.2 = x$; $x = 55.45$ lb; round off to tenths: 55.5 lb
> **Proof:** $1 \times 122 = 122$; $2.2 \times 55.45 = 121.99$ (rounds to 122)

Example 4: You have an injectable solution that is 50 mg strength. How many micrograms are in 50 mg?

> Equivalent: 1 mg = 1000 μg
> **Know**   **Want to Know**
> 1 mg : 1000 μg :: 50 mg : x μg
> $(1 \times x) = (1000 \times 50)$; $1x = 50,000$; $x = 50,000$; therefore, 50 mg = 50,000 μg
> **Proof:** $1 \times 50,000 = 50,000$; $1000 \times 50 = 50,000$

Example 5: Elixir is ordered as follows: "Give 2 tsp twice a day." How many milliliters would you give?

> Equivalent: 1 tsp = 5 ml
> **Know**   **Want to Know**
> 1 tsp : 5 ml :: 2 tsp : x ml
> $(1 \times x) = (5 \times 2)$; $1x = 10$; $x = 10$ ml
> **Proof:** $1 \times 10 = 10$; $5 \times 2 = 10$; $10 = 10$
> So, give 10 ml to equal 2 tsp.

Example 6: You have an injection that delivers 75 μg. How many milligrams does it deliver?

> Equivalent: 1 mg = 1000 μg
> **Know**   **Want to Know**
> 1 mg : 1000 μg :: x mg : 75 μg
> $(1 \times 75) = (1000 \times x)$; $75 = 1000x$; $x = 75/1000$; $x = 0.075$
> So, 75 μg = 0.075 mg. (*Don't forget the leading zero!*)
> Proof: $1 \times 75 = 75$; $1000 \times 0.075 = 75$; $75 = 75$

PRACTICE PROBLEMS

Calculate the following conversions using the information listed on page 147.

1. 600 mg = _____ μg

2. 1500 mg = _____ μg

3. 5000 μg = _____ mg

4. 5 g   = _____ mg

5. 2.5 g   = _____ mg

6. 900 mg = _____ g

7. 8 kg   = _____ g

8. 750 ml = _____ L

Copyright © 2002 by Mosby, Inc. All rights reserved.

9. 975 L   = _____ ml

10. 500 cc   = _____ L

11. gr xvi   = _____ mg

12. 90 mg   = _____ gr

13. 4 tsp   = _____ ml

14. 60 ml   = _____ tsp

15. 90 ml   = _____ tbsp

16. 3 oz   = _____ ml

17. 6 ml   = _____ oz

18. 90 kg   = _____ lb

19. 150 lb   = _____ kg

20. 11 kg   = _____ lb

SECTION II: CALCULATING ORAL DOSES

To calculate oral dosages of medications, use the same ratio and proportion procedures described in Section I. Label all terms, and check your answers by proving them.

The first step in doing medication dosage calculation problems is examining the order and the medication on hand. The units for both the order and the medicine on hand MUST be the same units (e.g., mg, ml). If they are not the same, then a conversion must first be done to change the ordered dose to the same units as the medication on hand.

Remember these rules:

- NEVER substitute one form of a medication for another, even if the dosage amount is the same. Parenteral forms of oral drugs are much stronger, and the results might be dangerous.
- Don't forget to place a zero in front of a decimal point (e.g., **0.**75 mg). It reminds you that the number is a decimal, not a whole number.
- Are the medication ordered and the medication on hand in the same units? If not, convert the drug ordered to the units of the drug at hand.
- Place what you have on hand (what you *know*)—information from the label—on the LEFT side of the equation.
- Place what is ordered (what you *want to know*) on the RIGHT side of the equation.
- Solve the equation as described in Section I.
- ALWAYS label the units of your answer (tablets, capsules, ml, etc).

Example 1: The prescription reads, "Give 500 mg PO." The unit dose is 250 mg/tablet. How many tablets will you give?

Ordered: 500 mg   **Unit dose:** 250 mg/tablet
NOTE: Units match (mg).

Know   *Want to Know*
250 mg : 1 tablet :: 500 mg : x tablet
$(250 \times x) = (1 \times 500)$; $250x = 500$; $x = 500/250 = 2$
Answer: Give 2 tablets.
Proof: $250 \times 2 = 500$; $1 \times 500 = 500$; $500 = 500$

Copyright © 2002 by Mosby, Inc. All rights reserved.

Example 2: The order is to give 175 mg. The tablets on hand are 350-mg scored tablets. How many tablets will you give?

Ordered: 175 mg　　　**Unit dose:** 350 mg/tablet
NOTE: Units match.

Know　　　　　　*Want to Know*
350 mg : 1 tablet :: 175 mg : x tablet
$(350 \times x) = (1 \times 175)$; $350x = 175$; $x = 175/350 = 0.5$
Answer: Give 0.5 tablet (one half of the scored tablet).
Proof: $350 \times 0.5 = 175$; $1 \times 175 = 175$; $175 = 175$

Example 3: You are asked to administer 100 mg of a drug. You have 0.05-g tablets on hand. How many tablets will you give?

Ordered: 100 mg　　　**Unit dose:** 0.05 g/tablet
NOTE: Units do not match.

First: Calculate: 100 mg = ? g (Equivalent: 1 g = 1000 mg)
Know　　　　*Want to Know*
1 g : 1000 mg :: x g : 100 mg
$(1 \times 100) = (1000 \times x)$; $100 = 1000x$; $x = 100/1000 = 0.1$
100 mg = 0.1 g

Now that you have the ordered dose and the dose on hand in the same units, you can complete the problem.
Ordered: 0.1 g (100 mg)　　　**Unit dose:** 0.05 g/tablet

Know　　*Want to Know*
0.05 g : 1 tablet :: 0.1g : x tablet
$(0.05 \times x) = (1 \times 0.1)$; $0.05x = 0.1$; $x = 0.1/0.05 = 2$
Answer: Give 2 tablets.
Proof: $0.05 \times 2 = 0.1$; $1 \times 0.1 = 0.1$; $0.1 = 0.1$

Example 4: You are instructed to give 0.5 g of a drug. You have 250-mg tablets on hand. How many tablets will you give?

Ordered: 0.5 g　　　**Unit dose**: 250 mg/tablet
NOTE: Units do not match.

First: Calculate: 0.5 g = ? mg (Equivalent: 1 g = 1000 mg)
Know　　　　*Want to Know*
1 g : 1000 mg :: 0.5 g : x mg
$(1 \times x) = (1000 \times 0.5)$; $1x = 500$; $x = 500$
0.5 g = 500 mg

Now that you have the ordered dose and the dose on hand in the same units, you can complete the problem.
Ordered: 500 mg (0.5 g)　　　**Unit dose:** 250 mg/tablet

Know　　　　　　*Want to Know*
250 mg : 1 tablet :: 500 mg : x tablet
$(250 \times x) = (1 \times 500)$; $250x = 500$; $x = 500/250 = 2$
Answer: Give 2 tablets.
Proof: $250 \times 2 = 500$; $1 \times 500 = 500$; $500 = 500$

Copyright © 2002 by Mosby, Inc. All rights reserved.

Example 5: You are to administer 200 mg of guaifenesin syrup. You have a bottle labeled 100 mg/5 ml. How many ml will you give?

Ordered: 200 mg   **Unit dose:** 100 mg/5ml
NOTE: Units match.

Know   *Want to Know*
100 mg : 5 ml :: 200 mg : x ml
$(100 \times x) = (5 \times 200)$; $100x = 1000$; $x = 1000/100 = 10$
Answer: Give 10 ml.
Proof: $100 \times 10 = 1000$; $5 \times 200 = 1000$; $1000 = 1000$

PRACTICE PROBLEMS

1. Dose ordered: ascorbic acid 0.5 g PO
   Dose on hand: 500-mg tablets
   How many tablets will you give? _____

2. Dose ordered: digoxin 0.5 mg PO
   Dose on hand: 250-mcg tablets
   How many tablets will you give? _____

3. Dose ordered: sulfisoxazole 0.25 g PO
   Dose on hand: 500-mg tablets
   How many tablets will you give? _____

4. Dose ordered: diphenhydramine elixir 50 mg PO
   Dose on hand: elixir 12.5 mg/5 ml
   How many milliliters will you give? _____

5. Dose ordered: aspirin 600 mg PO
   Dose on hand: gr v tablets
   How many tablets will you give? _____

6. Dose ordered: cefaclor 0.1 g PO
   Dose on hand: liquid 125 mg/5 ml
   How many milliliters will you give? _____

7. Dose ordered: quinidine sulfate 0.3 g PO
   Dose on hand: 100 mg tablets
   How many tablets will you give? _____

8. Dose ordered: potassium chloride elixir 30 mEq PO
   Dose on hand: 20 mEq/15ml
   How many milliliters will you give? _____

9. Dose ordered: Nembutal 0.15 g PO
   Dose on hand: 50 mg capsules
   How many capsules will you give? _____

10. Dose ordered: levodopa 2 g PO
    Dose on hand: 500 mg tablets
    How many tablets will you give? _____

SECTION III: RECONSTITUTING MEDICATIONS

Many medications come in powder or crystal form and must be reconstituted by the addition of a diluent to create a liquid form. Parenteral medications must be reconstituted before administration. Instructions for dissolving medications can be found in the literature that accompanies the medication or on the medication label. What will be given is the volume of the medication after it is dissolved in the diluent. For example, the instructions may read:

Add 1.2 ml normal saline to make 2 ml of reconstituted solution that yields 100 mg/ml.

This tells the user that the medication takes up 0.8 ml of space: 1.2 ml + 0.8 ml = 2 ml of medication solution. The label of the medication container will tell the user how many units, grams, milligrams, or micrograms are in each milliliter of the reconstituted drug. In this example, the dose on hand, after reconstitution, is 100 mg/ml.

Remember these rules:
- Read all instructions for reconstitution before doing anything! Be sure to ask a pharmacist if you have any questions.
- When reconstituting medications, be certain to use the exact *type* of diluent, and add the exact *amount* of diluent as directed. Substitutions or inaccurate amounts of diluent can inactivate the medication or alter the concentration, thus altering the dose received by the patient.

Copyright © 2002 by Mosby, Inc. All rights reserved.

- If the vial is a multiple-dose vial, the nurse who reconstitutes the medication must put the date, time, amount of diluent used, and his or her initials on the label.
- Many solutions are unstable after being reconstituted. Be sure to follow the directions on the label for proper storage of reconstituted medications.
- Make note of the time limit or expiration date for the reconstituted medication. Do not use the medication after it has expired.
- Ratio solutions indicate the number of grams of the medication per total milliliters of solution. For example, a medication that is designated 1:1000 has 1 g of medication per 1000 ml of solution.
- Percentage (%) solutions indicate the number of grams of the medication per 100 ml of solution. For example, a medication that is designated 10% has 10 g of drug per 100 ml of solution.
  COMPARE: "1:1000" indicates 1 g per 1000 ml
  　　　　　　　 "10%" indicates 10 g per 100 ml

As you calculate parenteral dosages:
- If the amount is greater than 1 ml, round x (the amount to be given) to tenths and use a 3-cc syringe to measure it.
- Small (less than 0.5 ml, or pediatric) dosages should be rounded to hundredths and measured in a tuberculin syringe. The tuberculin syringe is calibrated in 0.01-ml increments.
- THINK! For adults, the maximum volume of an intramuscular (IM) injection is usually 3 ml. Sometimes the dose might have to be given in two divided doses; for example, a dose of 4 ml IM would usually be divided into two 2-ml doses. However, if your calculations yield an unusual number, such as 10 ml IM, look over your calculation and repeat your math! Double-check your calculations with a peer.

Remember: Always note the route ordered—IM doses and IV doses are NOT always the same amount; confusing the route may have fatal results.

Example 1: You receive an order for morphine 10 mg IM. The medication vial reads: 8 mg/ml.
　How much morphine would you give?
　Does this medication require reconstitution?
　Would you use a 3-cc or a tuberculin syringe to measure this drug?
　Ordered: 10 mg　　　**Unit dose:** 8 mg/ml

Know　　　　　　　*Want to Know*
8 mg : 1 ml :: 10 mg : x ml
$(8 \times x) = (1 \times 10)$; $8x = 10$; $x = 10/8 = 1.25$, rounded to 1.3
Answer: 1.3 ml measured in a 3-cc syringe. This medication does not require reconstitution.
Proof: $8 \times 1.3 = 10.4$ (rounds to 10); $1 \times 10 = 10$

Example 2: The ordered dose is oxacillin 500 mg IV. The medication label reads:

> 500 mg OXACILLIN SODIUM FOR INJECTION
> For IM or IV use
> Add 2.7 ml sterile water for injection.
> Each 1.5 ml contains 250 mg oxacillin.

How much oxacillin would you give?
Does this medication require reconstitution?
Would you use a 3-cc or a tuberculin syringe to measure this drug?
Ordered: 500 mg　　　**Unit dose:** 250 mg/1.5 ml

Know　　　　　　　*Want to Know*
250 mg : 1.5 ml :: 500 mg : x ml
$(250 \times x) = (1.5 \times 500)$; $250x = 750$; $x = 750/250 = 3$
Answer: 3 ml measured in a 3-cc syringe. Reconstitute by adding 2.7 ml sterile water to the vial.
Proof: $250 \times 3 = 750$; $1.5 \times 500 = 750$; $750 = 750$

Copyright © 2002 by Mosby, Inc. All rights reserved.

Example 3: You receive an order for penicillin G potassium 400,000 U IM. The medication label reads:

| ONE MILLION UNITS |
| Penicillin G Potassium |
| |
| Use sterile saline as diluent as follows: |
| Add   Units per ml reconstituted solution |
| 18.2 ml   250,000 |
| 8.2 ml   500,000 |
| 3.2 ml   1,000,000 |

Which dilution would you choose for the ordered dose?
How much penicillin G potassium would you give?
Would you use a 3-cc or a tuberculin syringe to measure this drug?
Ordered: 400,000 U   **Unit dose:** Choosing the 8.2 diluent amount, the unit dose is 500,000/ml.

Know   *Want to Know*
500,000 U : 1 ml :: 400,000 : x ml
$(500,000 \times x) = (1 \times 400,000)$; $500,000x = 400,000$; $x = 400,000/500,000 = 0.8$
Answer: 0.8 ml measured in either a 3-cc or tuberculin syringe.
Proof: $500,000 \times 0.8 = 400,000$; $1 \times 400,000 = 400,000$; $400,000 = 400,000$
NOTE: Choose the concentration that is close to the ordered dose. Choosing the 8.2 diluent amount allows for the injection amount to be small yet easily measured. If you had chosen the 18.2 diluent amount, the injection would have been 1.6 ml; choosing the 3.2 diluent would have made the injection amount very small: 0.04 ml.

Example 4: You receive an order for epinephrine 0.6 mg SC. The medication label reads:

| 1 ml ampule |
| Epinephrine 1:1000 |
| For SC or IM use |

What is the dose on hand?
How much epinephrine would you give?
Would you use a 3-cc or a tuberculin syringe to measure the drug?

First: Figure the dose on hand.
1:1000 = 1 g in 1000 ml = 1000 mg in 1000 ml = **1 mg in 1 ml**

Then complete the problem:
Ordered: 0.6 mg   **Unit dose:** 1 mg/ml

Know   *Want to Know*
1 mg : 1 ml :: 0.6 mg : x ml
$(1 \times x) = (1 \times 0.6)$; $1x = 0.6$; $x = 0.6$
Answer: 0.6 ml measured in either a 3-cc or tuberculin syringe.
Proof: $1 \times 0.6 = 0.6$; $1 \times 0.6 = 0.6$; $0.6 = 0.6$

Copyright © 2002 by Mosby, Inc. All rights reserved.

Example 5: Magnesium sulfate 5 g IV over 3 hours is the dosage ordered. The medication label reads:

> 10 ml vial
> Magnesium Sulfate 10%
> For IM or IV use

What is the dose on hand?
How much magnesium sulfate would you give?

First: Figure the dose on hand.
10% = 10 g in 100 ml = **0.1 g per 1 ml**

Then complete the problem:
Ordered: 5 g   **Unit dose:** 0.1 g/ml

Know   *Want to Know*
0.1 g : 1 ml :: 5 g : x ml
$(0.1 \times x) = (1 \times 5)$; $0.1x = 5$; $x = 5/0.1$; $x = 50$
Answer: 50 ml
Proof: $0.1 \times 50 = 5$; $1 \times 5 = 5$; $5 = 5$

PRACTICE PROBLEMS

1. Dose ordered: thiamine 200 mg
   On hand: 10-ml vial, 100 mg/ml
   How much will you give? _____

2. Dose ordered: gentamicin 60 mg IM
   On hand: 40 mg/ml
   How much will you give? _____

3. Dose ordered: heparin 8000 U SC
   On hand: 1-ml vial, 10,000 U/ml
   How much will you give? _____

4. Dose ordered: methicillin 750 mg IV
   On hand: 1-g vial
   Instructions for reconstitution: Add 1.5 ml
   sterile water. Reconstituted solution will contain approximately 500 mg methicillin solution
   per ml.
   How much will you give? _____

5. Dose ordered: ampicillin 500 mg IV
   On hand: 1 g vial
   Instructions for reconstitution: Add 66 ml ster-
   ile water. Reconstituted solution will contain
   125 mg/5 ml.
   How much will you give? _____

6. Dose ordered: penicillin G potassium 300,000
   U IM.
   On hand: 1,000,000-U vial
   Instructions for reconstitution: Using only ster-
   ile water, add 9.6 ml to provide 100,000 U/ml,
   or 4.6 ml to provide 200,000 U/ml.
   Which concentration would you choose for
   this dose? _____
   How much will you give? _____

7. Dose ordered: epinephrine 750 µg SC
   On hand: 1:1000
   How much will you give? _____

8. Dose ordered: Isuprel 0.2 mg
   On hand: 1:5000
   How much will you give? _____

9. Dose ordered: calcium gluconate 900 mg
   On hand: calcium gluconate 10%, 100-ml vial
   How much will you give? _____

10. Dose ordered: magnesium sulfate 4 g
    On hand: magnesium sulfate 50%, 10-ml vial
    How much will you give? _____

Copyright © 2002 by Mosby, Inc. All rights reserved.

SECTION IV: PEDIATRIC CALCULATIONS

Doses used in pediatric patients must differ from those used in adults. The most common method for calculating doses for pediatric patients is weight-based, i.e., mg/kg. However, several formulas for calculating drug doses in young patients have been developed. See Chapter 3 in your text for a description of Clark's rule (based on weight, for children older than 2 years); Young's rule (based on age, for children older than 2 years); and Fried's rule (based on age, for children younger than 1 year).

Body Surface Area Calculations

The body surface area (BSA) is a common method used to calculate therapeutic pediatric dosages. It requires the use of a chart called a nomogram (see Figure 3-1 in your text) that converts weight to square meters (m^2) of BSA. The average adult is assumed to weigh 140 lb and have a BSA of 1.73 m^2. The BSA may be used to calculate the pediatric dose of certain medications.

- For a child of normal height and weight, find the m^2 for that weight on the shaded area of the nomogram chart.
  Example: Using Figure 3-1 in your text, find the BSA for a child who weighs 40 lb and is 38 inches tall (normal height for her weight). According to the nomogram, the BSA for 40 lb is 0.74 m^2.

- For a child who is underweight or overweight, the surface area is indicated at the point where a straight line connecting the height and weight intersects the unshaded surface area (SA) column.
  Example: Using Figure 3-1, find the BSA for a child who weighs 25 lb and has a height of 30 inches (underweight). According to the nomogram, the BSA for this child is 0.51 m^2.

There are two types of BSA problems.

➤ The first type involves medications for which the literature provides recommended dosages in m^2.

STEP 1: Check the order, and look up the recommended dose.
The order is for 15 mg PO.
The literature states that 40 mg/m^2 is safe for children.

STEP 2: Determine child's height and weight. Then consult the appropriate nomogram to obtain the BSA in m^2. This child weighs 22 lb and has a normal height of 70 cm. The BSA is approximately 0.46 m^2.

STEP 3: Calculate the recommended mg/m^2 dose (from the literature) using ratio and proportion. Then, for a safety check, compare it with the dose ordered.
For this calculation, what you *know* is the literature's recommendation (40 mg/m^2). What you *want to know* is the milligrams per the child's BSA (which is 0.46 m^2).
Know   ***Want to Know***
40 mg : 1 m^2 :: x mg : 0.46 m^2
$(40 \times 0.46) = (1 \times x)$; $18.4 = 1x$; $x = 18.4$ (Pediatric doses are rounded to tenths place; *do not* round to whole numbers.)
Answer: 18.4 mg is the safe dose limit.
Decision: The order for 15 mg is safe.

Practice:
The medication ordered is 100 mg.

STEP 1: The literature recommends 50 mg/m^2 for children.

STEP 2: The child weighs 10 lb and has a normal height for his weight. The BSA is 0.27 m^2.

Copyright © 2002 by Mosby, Inc. All rights reserved.

STEP 3: Calculate the dose for this child's BSA:
Know   *Want to Know*
50 mg : 1 m^2 :: *x* mg : 0.27 m^2
$(50 \times 0.27) = (1 \times x)$; $13.5 = 1x$; $x = 13.5$ (Pediatric doses are rounded to tenths place; *do not* round to whole numbers.)
Answer: 13.5 mg is the safe dose limit.
Decision: The order for 15 mg exceeds the safe dose limit and therefore is NOT safe. Notify the physician.

➤ The second type of BSA involves situations when a recommended dose for adults is cited in the literature, but not for children.

STEP 1: Determine the BSA (m^2) of the child by dividing the adult dose by 1.73 m^2 (the average adult's BSA—remember?).

STEP 2: Multiply the result by the average adult dose.

$$\frac{\text{Child's BSA (m}^2)}{\text{Average adult's BSA}} \times \text{Average adult dose of drug } = \text{ Estimated child's dose}$$

Example: A 6-lb child has a BSA of 0.20 m^2, and the average adult dose of a drug is 300 mg. What would be the estimated safe dose for a child?
$$\frac{0.20 \text{ m}^2}{1.73 \text{ m}^2} \times 300 \text{ mg} = 34.68 \text{ mg}$$
Answer: 34.7 mg is the estimated safe dose for this child. (Round to tenths place for pediatric doses.)

Practice:
The average adult dose for a medication is 20 mg. The child has a BSA of 0.60 m^2.
What would be the estimated safe dose for a child?
$$\frac{0.60 \text{ m}^2}{1.73 \text{ m}^2} \times 20 \text{ mg} = 6.94 \text{ mg}$$
Answer: 6.9 mg is the estimated safe dose for this child. (Round to tenths place for pediatric doses.)

Weight-Based Calculations

When calculating the proper dose according to weight, **STEP 1** involves changing the weight from pounds to kilograms (if necessary).
- Be careful when converting ounces and pounds to kilograms. First, ounces must be converted to part of a pound (by dividing the ounces by 16). Remember, 16 ounces = 1 pound. Therefore, 8 oz does not convert to 0.8 lb! Convert 8 ounces to pounds by dividing by 16: 8/16 = 0.5; 8 oz = 0.5 lb.
- Once you have converted ounces to pounds, then add the ounces to the pounds. For example, 10 lb 8 oz would equal 10.5 lb. You are now ready to convert pounds to kilograms.
- Remember: 1 kg = 2.2 lb. To convert 10.5 lb to kilograms, divide the pounds by 2.2.
  1 kg : 2.2 lb :: *x* kg : 10.5 lb; $(1 \times 10.5) = (2.2 \times x)$; $10.5 = 2.2x$; $x = 10.5/2.2 = 4.8$ kg (rounded to tenths)
- DO NOT round pediatric weights to whole numbers!
Once you have converted the child's weight to kg, you are ready for STEP 2.

STEP 2 involves calculating the therapeutic dosage ranges for a child based on his or her weight. The nurse uses the child's weight (in kilograms) to calculate the low and high acceptable doses for that medication. This will give a range of dosage that this child could receive for this medication.

STEP 3 involves THINKING and comparing the ordered dose with the therapeutic range that was calculated for that child. If the ordered dose is under or over the calculated therapeutic range, then do not give the medication and notify the physician.

Copyright © 2002 by Mosby, Inc. All rights reserved.

- **STEP 1:** Convert the child's weight from pounds to kilograms.

- **STEP 2:** Calculate therapeutic dose range (low and high).

- **STEP 3:**   (1)   Is the ordered dose safe (does not exceed the dosage range)?
                  (2)   Is the ordered dose therapeutic (falling within the recommended dosage range, not too low)?

Example 1: The ordered dose is 50 mg acetaminophen. The child weighs 15 lb. The therapeutic range for acetaminophen is 10 to 15 mg/kg/dose.

STEP 1: Convert pounds to kilograms by dividing 15 by 2.2.
15/2.2 = 6.82; 15 lb = 6.8 kg (Do not round pediatric weights to whole numbers.)

STEP 2: Calculate the therapeutic range for this child based on his weight.
Low dose: 10 mg/kg/dose × 6.8 kg = 68 mg/dose
High dose: 15 mg/kg/dose × 6.8 kg = 102 mg/dose
The therapeutic range for this child is 68 to 102 mg/dose for acetaminophen.

STEP 3: Compare the ordered dose with the therapeutic range calculated in STEP 2.
Answer: The ordered dose of 50 mg is not therapeutic because it falls under the low recommended dose.

If the doctor orders 110 mg of acetaminophen for this child, would that be a safe and therapeutic dose?
Answer: No, it would neither be safe nor therapeutic because it is higher than 102 mg.

Example 2: The ordered dose is amoxicillin 275 mg q8hr PO. The patient weighs 35 lb. The therapeutic range for amoxicillin is 20 to 50 mg/kg/24 hr.

STEP 1: Convert pounds to kilograms by dividing 35 by 2.2.
35/2.2 = 15.9; 35 lb = 15.9 kg

STEP 2: Calculate the therapeutic range for this child based on his weight.
Low dose: 20 mg/kg/24 hr × 15.9 kg = 318 mg/24 hr
High dose: 50 mg/kg/24 hr × 15.9 kg = 795 mg/24 hr
NOTE: These ranges are for 24 hours! The dosage is every 8 hours, so dividing 24 hours by 8 tells us that there will be 3 doses within 24 hours. To figure out the single dosage for the low and high ranges, divide each 24-hour dose by 3:
318 mg/24 hr divided by 3 doses = 106 mg/dose
795 mg/24 hr divided by 3 doses = 265 mg/dose
Answer: The safe range for a single dose of amoxicillin for this child is 106 to 265 mg/dose.

(An alternate way to figure the safe range for a single dose is to calculate the amount of medication the ordered dose would provide in 24 hours. In this example, knowing there are 3 doses given every 8 hours in a 24-hour period, multiplying the dose ordered by 3 would yield the ordered dose for 24 hours: 275 mg × 3 doses = 825 mg/24 hr.)

STEP 3: Is the ordered dose of 275 mg therapeutic for this child?
Answer: No, the ordered dose of 275 mg exceeds the therapeutic range for this patient. Consult the physician. (Note also that the calculated 24-hour dose of 825 mg/24 hr exceeds the high range of 795 mg/24 hr calculated for this child.)

Many pediatric medications come in several concentrations. It is ESSENTIAL to use the correct concentration of medication to ensure accurate dosage and prevent accidental underdosage or overdosage.

Copyright © 2002 by Mosby, Inc. All rights reserved.

Example: Acetaminophen comes in many forms:
        drops, 80 mg/0.8 ml
        elixir, 80, 120, or 160 mg/5 ml
        suspension, 160 mg/5 ml
        chewable tablet, 80 or 160 mg/tablet
        tablet, 325, 500, or 650 mg/tablet
        suppository, 80, 120, 125, 325, or 650 mg

A 4-month-old child weighs 13 lb and has a fever of 101.5° F. What would be the therapeutic range of acetaminophen this infant could receive?

STEP 1: 13 lb = 5.9 kg

STEP 2: Low dose: 10 mg/kg/dose × 5.9 = 59 mg/dose
         High dose: 15 mg/kg/dose × 5.9 = 88.5 mg/dose
Answer: The therapeutic range for this infant is 59 to 88.5 mg/dose.
Referring to the forms of acetaminophen listed above, which form would you choose if this infant was to receive an 80-mg dose?
Answer: Choose the drops, 80 mg/0.8 ml, and administer 0.8 ml with a calibrated oral syringe or dropper.

PRACTICE PROBLEMS

1. Your 6-year-old patient weighs 40 lb. Morphine sulfate via continuous infusion is ordered at 1 mg/hr. The therapeutic range for continuous IV infusion is 0.025 to 2 mg/kg/hr.
   a. What are the low and high doses for this child? _____
   b. Is the ordered dose within a safe and therapeutic range? _____

2. A 5-year-old weighs 33 lb. Ibuprofen is ordered at 120 mg PO q8hr. The therapeutic range is 5 to 10 mg/kg/dose q6hr to q8hr, and the maximum dose is 40 mg/kg/24 hr.
   a. What are the low and high doses for this child? _____
   b. What is the maximum amount this child can receive in 24 hours? _____
   c. Is the ordered dose within a safe and therapeutic range? _____

3. A 10-year-old patient weighs 70 lb. Fortraz is ordered at 1.7 g q8hr IV. The therapeutic range is 90 to 150 mg/kg/24 hr (divided q8hr IV).
   a. What are the low and high doses for this child in 24 hours? _____
   b. What are the low and high doses for this child per individual dose? _____
   c. Is the ordered dose within a safe and therapeutic range? _____

4. Your patient weighs 15 lb. The medication ordered is 150 μg bid. The therapeutic range of the medication is 0.02 to 0.05 mg/kg/day.
   a. What are the low and high doses for this child in 24 hours? _____
   b. What are the low and high doses for this child per individual dose? _____
   c. Is the ordered dose within a safe and therapeutic range? _____

5. A child weighs 34 lb. The medication ordered is 30 mg IM preoperatively. The therapeutic range is 1 to 2.2 mg/kg.
   a. What are the low and high doses for this child per individual dose? _____
   b. Is the ordered dose within a safe and therapeutic range? _____

6. For a child weighing 50 lb, medication is ordered at 0.1 mg daily IV. The therapeutic range is 4 to 5 mcg/kg/day.
   a. What are the low and high doses for this child per individual dose? _____
   b. Is the ordered dose within a safe and therapeutic range? _____

Copyright © 2002 by Mosby, Inc. All rights reserved.

SECTION V: BASIC INTRAVENOUS CALCULATIONS

Intravenous (IV) fluids and medications are given over a designated period of time. For instance, the order may read:

> *Give 1000 ml normal saline over 8 hours IV.*

For IVs that infuse with an infusion pump, the milliliters per hour is calculated (ml/hr).
For IVs that infuse by gravity, the rate at which an IV is given is measured in terms of *drops per minute* (gtt/min).

To calculate ml/hr and gtt/min, we need to consider what the order contains and what equipment is used. In order to calculate drops per minute we need to know the drop factor of the IV tubing. The size of the drops delivered per milliliter can vary with different types of tubing. The drop factor of a certain tubing set is printed on the label.
Adding to the above order:

> *The drop factor for the IV tubing is 15 gtt/ml.*

The order now reads:

> *Give 1000 ml normal saline over 8 hours IV. The drop factor is 15 gtt/ml.*

STEP 1: Calculate milliliters per hour.
We *know* that 1000 ml is to infuse over 8 hours. We *want to know* how much is to infuse over 1 hour.
   Set up the equation:

Know   ***Want to Know***

1000 ml : 8 hr :: x ml : 1 hr
$(1000 \times 1) = (8 \times x)$; $1000 = 8x$; $x = 8/1000$; $x = 125$ ml/hr
Rate: To give 1000 ml normal saline over 8 hours, give 125 ml/hr for 8 hours.
A quick way to determine the hourly rate is to divide the TOTAL VOLUME by the TOTAL TIME (if the time is in hours): 1000 ml ÷ 8 hr = 125 ml/hr.

STEP 2: Calculate the gtt/min.
To set up a gravity IV drip, further calculations are needed. To ensure the proper rate, one must count the drops per minute (gtt/min).
We know the rate is 125 ml/hr and the drop factor is 15 gtt/ml. Since we need to change from *hours* to *minutes*, another equivalent we'll need is 60 min = 1 hr.
When ml/hr is known, the formula for calculating gtt/min is as follows:

$$\frac{\text{drop factor (gtt/ml)}}{\text{time (min)}} \times \text{hourly rate (ml/hr)} = \text{gtt/min}$$

Plugging in what we know:

$$\frac{15 \text{ gtt/ml*}}{60 \text{ min/hr}} \times 125 \text{ ml/hr} = x \text{ gtt/min}$$

*To make it easier to calculate, reduce the 15/60 fraction to 1/4 before multiplying by 125.
$1/4 \times 125 = 125/4 = 31.25$ (round ml/hr to whole numbers)
Answer: 31 gtt/min for a gravity drip

Points to remember:
- The drop factor varies per IV tubing set manufacturer. It can range from 10 to 20 gtt/min.
- Infusion sets that deliver 60 gtt/min are called microdrips.
- **STEP 1:** To calculate ml/hr, divide the TOTAL VOLUME by the TOTAL TIME (in hours).
- **STEP 2:** To calculate gtt/min when the hourly rate is known, use the formula:
  $$\frac{\text{drop factor (gtt/ml)}}{\text{time (min)}} \times \text{hourly rate (ml/hr)} = \text{gtt/min}$$
- THINK! If you are using an infusion pump, you need to calculate milliliters per hour.
- THINK! Round off your answer to the nearest whole number. You cannot count a partial drop! Also, IV electronic infusion pumps will usually use the nearest whole number in ml.

Copyright © 2002 by Mosby, Inc. All rights reserved.

Example 1: The order reads "200 ml to be infused for 1 hr." If the drop factor is 15 gtt/ml, how many gtt/min will be given?
Start at STEP 1 or STEP 2?
STEP 1: Calculate ml/hr. Divide total volume by the total time (in hours).
200 ml over 1 hr = 200 ml/hr.
STEP 2: Calculate gtt/min using the formula:
$$\frac{drop\ factor}{time\ (min)} \times hourly\ rate = 15/60 \times 200 = 1/4 \times 200 = 50$$

Answer: 50 gtt/min

Example 2: The order is for 1000 ml to infuse at 150 ml/hr. The drop factor is 20 gtt/ml. How many gtt/min will be given?
Start at STEP 1 or STEP 2?
Start at STEP 2. The hourly rate, 150 ml/hr, has been given.
STEP 2: Calculate gtt/min using the formula:
$$\frac{drop\ factor}{time\ (min)} \times hourly\ rate = 20/60 \times 150 = 1/3 \times 150 = 50$$

Answer: 50 gtt/min

Example 3: You receive an order for 200 ml to be infused for 90 minutes. You have a microdrip set (60 gtt/ml). How many gtt/min will be given?
Start at STEP 1 or STEP 2?
Start at STEP 1. Calculate the hourly rate. Remember, 60 min = 1 hr.
STEP 1:
Know   **Want to Know**
200 ml : 90 min :: x ml : 60 min
$(200 \times 60) = (90 \times x)$; $12,000 = 90x$; $x = 12,000/90$; $x = 133.33$
Rate: 133 ml/hr (*Round to nearest whole number.*)
STEP 2: Calculate gtt/min using the formula:
$$\frac{drop\ factor}{time\ (min)} \times hourly\ rate = 60/60 \times 133 = 1 \times 133 = 133$$

Answer: 133 gtt/min
Short cut: For microdrips, when the drip factor is 60 and the time is 60 minutes, the "60's" cancel out to "1" and the result is that the ordered ml/hr = the gtt/min.

PRACTICE PROBLEMS

Calculate the following, and prove your answers:

1. Give 1000 ml lactated Ringer's solution over 6 hours. The drop factor is 15 gtt/ml.
   Start at STEP 1 or STEP 2?
   a. ml/hr: _____
   b. gtt/min: _____

2. Infuse 600 ml blood over 3 hours. The blood administration set has a drop factor of 10 gtt/ml.
   Start at STEP 1 or STEP 2?
   a. ml/hr: _____
   b. gtt/min: _____

3. Infuse 1000 ml normal saline over 12 hours, using tubing with a drop factor of 15 gtt/ml.
   Start at STEP 1 or STEP 2?
   a. ml/hr: _____
   b. gtt/min: _____

4. Infuse 200 ml D_5NS over 2 hours using a microdrip set.
   Start at STEP 1 or STEP 2?
   a. ml/hr: _____
   b. gtt/min: _____
   c. What is the drop factor? _____

Copyright © 2002 by Mosby, Inc. All rights reserved.

5. Infuse D$_5$W at 75 ml/hr. The drop factor is 10 gtt/ml. *Start at STEP 1 or STEP 2?*
gtt/min: _____

6. Infuse D$_5$W at 75 ml/hr. The drop factor is 15 gtt/ml. *Start at STEP 1 or STEP 2?*
gtt/min: _____

7. Infuse D$_5$W at 75 ml/hr. The drop factor is 20 gtt/ml. *Start at STEP 1 or STEP 2?*
gtt/min: _____

8. After looking at your answers for questions 5, 6, and 7, what observation can you make about the relationship between the drop factor and the resulting gtt/min?

9. Give 50 ml of an antibiotic over 30 minutes. You will be using an infusion pump.
Start at STEP 1 or STEP 2?
   a. ml/hr: _____
   b. gtt/min: _____
   c. Do you need to calculate both ml/hr and gtt/min for this situation? _____

10. Infuse 500 ml normal saline over 4 hours, using tubing with a drop factor of 60 gtt/ml. *Start at STEP 1 or STEP 2?*
   a. ml/hr: _____
   b. gtt/min: _____

PRACTICE QUIZ

Convert the following:

1. 750 μg = _____ mg

2. 8 g = _____ mg

3. 250 lb = _____ kg

4. 75 kg = _____ lb

5. 3 tsp = _____ ml

6. gr x = _____ mg

Calculate the following, and prove your answers:

7. Dose ordered: indomethacin (oral suspension) 50 mg qid
Dose on hand: Oral suspension 25 mg/ml
How much would you give per dose?
_____

8. Dose ordered: procainamide 0.5 g q4hr
Dose on hand: 500-mg tablets.
How much would you give per dose?
_____

9. Dose ordered: phenytoin 100 mg IV now
Dose on hand: 5-ml ampule labeled "50 mg/ml"
How much would you give per dose?
_____

10. Dose ordered: lidocaine 50 mg IV now
Dose on hand: lidocaine 1% in 5-ml ampule
How much would you give? _____

11. Dose ordered: epinephrine 0.25 mg SC now
Dose on hand: epinephrine 1:1000 ampule
How much would you give? _____

12. Dose ordered: heparin 15,000 U IV bolus
Dose on hand: heparin 10,000 U/ml (5-ml vial)
How much would you give? _____

13. Dose ordered: polythiazide 1 mg PO daily
Dose on hand: polythiazide 1-mg tablet
Child's weight: 22 lb
Therapeutic range: 0.02 to 0.08 mg/kg once daily
   a. What is the safe and therapeutic range for this child? _____
   b. Is the ordered dose safe and therapeutic?
   _____

14. Ordered: Infuse normal saline 500 ml over 8 hours. The tubing drop factor is 15.
   a. What is the rate of the IV? _____
   b. What is the gtt/min? _____

15. Ordered: D$_5$1/2 normal saline to infuse at 50 ml/hr via an infusion pump.
   a. How will this be administered—ml/hr or gtt/min? _____
   b. What is the rate? _____

Copyright © 2002 by Mosby, Inc. All rights reserved.

16. Ordered: 1000 ml D$_5$W to infuse over 24 hours. The tubing drop factor is 60.
    a. What is the rate of the IV? _____
    b. What is the gtt/min? _____

17. Ordered: cephalothin 500 mg IVPB q6hr.
    Dose on hand: cephalothin powder for injection (See label.)

    > 1 g vial
    > CEPHALOTHIN
    > Add 5 ml sterile water for injection.
    > Solution will contain 200 mg/ml.

    a. How much does this vial contain?

        _____

    b. How much will you give for each dose?

        _____

18. Ordered: penicillin G 200,000 U IM qid
    Dose on hand: penicillin G 5,000,000 U
    The medication label reads:

    > FIVE MILLION UNITS multidose vial
    > Penicillin G
    >
    > Use sterile saline as diluent as follows:
    >
    > | Add | Units per ml reconstituted solution |
    > | --- | --- |
    > | 23 ml | 200,000 |
    > | 18 ml | 250,000 |
    > | 8 ml | 500,000 |
    > | 3 ml | 1,000,000 |

    a. What concentration should you choose?

        _____

    b. How much sterile saline should you add to the vial to obtain this concentration?

        _____

    c. How much medication will you give?

        _____

    d. How do you label the vial? _____

19. A child weighs 31 lb.
    Dose ordered: ceftriaxone sodium 600 mg IV q12hr
    Dose on hand: See label.
    Safe dose range: Up to 100 mg/kg/day in 2 divided doses

    > 1 g
    > ceftriaxone sodium
    > DIRECTIONS: Add 9.6 ml sterile water for injection to equal 100 mg/ml.

    a. How much would you give for this dose?

        _____

    b. What is the safe dose range for this child (in 24 hours)? _____
    c. What is the safe dose range for this child (per dose)? _____
    d. Is the ordered dose within a safe and therapeutic range? _____

20. Dose ordered: digoxin 125 μg daily
    Dose on hand: Pediatric elixir 0.05 mg/ml
    How much would you give? _____

Copyright © 2002 by Mosby, Inc. All rights reserved.

Answers

Copyright © 2002 by Mosby, Inc. All rights reserved.

WORKSHEETS

CHAPTER 1
The Nursing Process and Drug Therapy

1. c
2. d
3. c
4. b
5. a
6. S, O, O, O, S, S
7. Answers may vary slightly with each one but should include: **Right drug:** Compare drug orders and medication labels. Consider whether the drug is appropriate for that patient. Obtain information about the patient regarding his or her past and present medical history and a thorough, updated medication history, including OTC medications. **Right dose:** Check the order and the label on the medication, and check for all of the five rights at least three times before administering the medication. Recheck the math calculations for dosages, and contact the physician when clarification is needed. **Right time:** Assess for a conflict between the pharmacokinetic and pharmacodynamic properties of the drugs prescribed and the patient's lifestyle and likelihood of compliance. **Right route:** Never assume the route for administration or change it; always check with the physician or prescriber. **Right patient:** Check the patient's identity before administering a medication. Ask for the patient's name, and check the identification band or bracelet to confirm the patient's name, ID number, age, and allergies.
8. a. specific health status
   b. specific problems, defined as alterations in human needs
   c. plans to solve the problems
   d. assessment
   e. objective
   f. subjective
   g. analyze
   h. goals
   i. outcome criteria
   j. implementation
   k. evaluation

9. To avoid medication errors: *Follow the five rights!* Carefully read all labels for the five rights of medication administration. Repeat a verbal order, and spell the drug name out loud. *Never* assume a route of administration; if an order is unclear or incomplete, clarify the order with the prescriber. *Always* read the label three times, and check the medication order before administering the medication. See text for other possible answers. If a medication error occurs: Reporting medication errors is a professional responsibility. Report the error following the institution's policies and procedures. In addition, report the medication error through the United States Pharmacopoeia Medication Errors Reporting Program (USP-MERP).

CHAPTER 2
Pharmacologic Principles

1. d
2. c
3. b
4. d
5. a
6. b
7. i
8. j
9. f
10. g
11. a
12. h
13. d
14. e
15. c
16. Because muscles have a greater blood supply than the skin, drugs injected intramuscularly are typically absorbed faster than those injected subcutaneously. Absorption can be increased by applying heat to the injection site or by massaging it, which increases the blood flow to the area, thus enhancing absorption.

163

CHAPTER 3
Lifespan Considerations

1. c
2. a
3. d
4. b
5. a
6. d
7. b
8. e
9. a
10. c
11. More than 80% of all elderly patients have one or more chronic illnesses. They may see several different specialists, who may each prescribe their own sets of medications. In addition, some patients self-administer OTC products to ease the discomfort of even more ailments. This practice is called *polypharmacy*.
12. Based on Table 3-3, students may choose a variety of conditions affecting the cardiovascular, gastrointestinal, hepatic, and renal systems.

CHAPTER 4
Legal, Ethical, and Cultural Considerations

1. b
2. a
3. d
4. c
5. b
6. d
7. a
8. c
9. b
10. c
11. a
12. d
13. b
14. Answers will vary, depending on the group identified.
   a. Barriers may include language, poverty, access, pride, and beliefs regarding medical practices.
   b. Attitudes will vary depending on the groups identified.
   c. Questions may include the following topics: health beliefs and practices, past use of medicine, folk remedies, home remedies, use of nonprescription drugs, OTC treatments, usual responses to illness, responsiveness to medical treatments, religious practices and beliefs, and dietary habits.

CHAPTER 5
Patient Education and Drug Therapy

1. Students should refer to the information in Chapter 23 ("Antihypertensive Agents") for specific information about antihypertensive drug therapy. In addition, the students who are assigned to the 78-year-old patient should also use the strategies described in Box 5-2, "Selected Aging Changes and Educational Strategies Appropriate to Pharmacology Content."
2. Refer to Box 5-3, "General Teaching Principles." Some strategies include using pictures and illustrations, demonstrating by example, and finding an interpreter.
3. a. Answers will vary, but this nursing diagnosis should address a knowledge deficit.
   b. Answers will vary, but this nursing diagnosis should address noncompliance.
4. Answers will vary, depending on the type of medication. Refer to the appropriate chapters for specific patient/family teaching and possible goals/expected outcomes.
5. Teaching plans will vary somewhat in format, but each should contain the following information:
   a. Assessment items should include some of the items listed in the text under the heading "Assessment of Learning Need Related to Drug Therapy."
   b. A "Deficient Knowledge" nursing diagnosis.
   c. A measurable goal with outcome criteria related to the nursing diagnosis.
   d. Specific educational strategies for providing the information needed.
   e. Specific questions designed to validate whether learning has occurred.

CHAPTER 6
Over-the-Counter Drugs and Herbal Remedies

Critical Thinking Crossword

Across
1. Kava
4. Ephedra
8. Garlic
10. Saw palmetto
11. Herbs

Down
2. Aloe
3. Prozac
5. Echinacea

Copyright © 2002 by Mosby, Inc. All rights reserved.

6. Gingko
7. Ginseng
9. Legend

Multiple-choice and short answer

1. c
2. a
3. b
4. c
5. d
6. d
7. NSAIDs, histamine-blocking agents, garlic, gingko, and ginseng

CHAPTER 7
Substance Abuse

1. h
2. i
3. f
4. e
5. g
6. d
7. j
8. a
9. c
10. b
11. c
12. d
13. a
14. c
15. b
16. The nicotine transdermal system (patch) and nicotine polacrilex (gum) can be used to provide nicotine without the carcinogens in tobacco. The patches use a stepwise reduction in delivery, and work by gradually reducing the nicotine dose over time. With use of the gum, rapid chewing releases an immediate dose of nicotine, but this dose is about half of what the average smoker receives from one cigarette, and the onset of action is longer than with smoking. Therefore the reinforcement and self-reward effects of smoking are minimized. Bupropion (Zyban) is an antidepressant and is the first nicotine-free prescription medicine used to treat nicotine dependence.

CHAPTER 8
Photo Atlas of Drug Administration

1. b
2. c
3. a
4. b
5. c

6. c
7. b
8. a
9. c
10. c
11. b
12. d
13. a
14. a
15. d
16. a. Palpate sites for masses or tenderness.
    b. Note the integrity and size of the muscle and palpate for tenderness.
    c. Note any lesions or discolorations of the forearm.
17. a. For an average-sized patient: spread the skin tightly across the injection site or pinch the skin with the nondominant hand. Inject the needle quickly and firmly at a 45- to 90-degree angle, then release the skin if it was pinched. For an obese patient: pinch the skin at the site, and inject the needle below the tissue fold.
    b. Position the nondominant hand at the proper anatomic landmarks, and spread the skin tightly. Inject the needle quickly into the muscle at a 90-degree angle. If the patient's muscle mass is small, grasp the body of the muscle between the thumb and other fingers. If the medication is irritating, use the Z-track method.
    c. With the nondominant hand, stretch the skin over the site with the forefinger or thumb. With the needle almost against the patient's skin, insert it slowly at a 5- to 15-degree angle until resistance is felt; then advance the needle through the epidermis to approximately 3 mm below the surface. The needle tip can be seen through skin.
18. Remove the needle, discard the medication and syringe, and repeat the procedure.
19. Rather than pouring it into a medication cup, draw volumes of less than 10 ml in a syringe (without the needle).

CHAPTER 9
Analgesic Agents

Critical Thinking Crossword

Across
2. Agonist
6. Superficial
7. Pain tolerance
10. Threshold
12. Opioid
13. Partial

Copyright © 2002 by Mosby, Inc. All rights reserved.

14. Abstinence

Down
1. Antagonist
3. Chronic
4. Visceral
5. Opiate
6. Somatic
8. Acute
9. Compulsive
11. Adjuvant

Multiple-choice and matching

1. b
2. d
3. c
4. d
5. d
6. g
7. f
8. i
9. h
10. d
11. b
12. j
13. c
14. a
15. e

CHAPTER 10
General and Local Anesthetics

Critical Thinking Crossword

Across
3. Pancuronium
6. General
7. Topical
8. Adjunctive
9. Local

Down
1. Atropine
2. Anesthetics
3. Parenteral
4. Balanced
5. Regional

Multiple-choice and short answer

1. d
2. b
3. a
4. b
5. c
6. c

7. Pediatric patients are more susceptible to problems such as CNS depression, toxicity, atelectasis, pneumonia, and cardiac abnormalities because their hepatic, cardiac, respiratory, and renal systems are not fully developed or fully functional.
8. These agents cause paralysis, but not anesthesia. The patient is still able to hear you and feel your touch. It is important to remain professional at all times and to take the time to orient the patient to his surroundings, to what noises mean, and to what you are going to be doing to him.

CHAPTER 11
Central Nervous System Depressants and Muscle Relaxants

1. a
2. b
3. a
4. d
5. c
6. Answers should reflect the discussion under "Toxicity and Overdose" on p. 160 of the text.
7. These agents can be used for insomnia only if they are limited to short-term use (less than 2 to 4 weeks). With long-term use, rebound insomnia and severe withdrawal can develop.
8. Geriatric patients should be started on lower doses because they generally experience a more pronounced effect from benzodiazepines.
9. a. Ask about allergies, CNS disorders, sleep disorders, diabetes, addictive disorders, personality disorders, thyroid conditions, and renal and liver function status.
   b. Alcohol, CNS depressants, and other prescribed or OTC medications.
   c. The patient's age matters because of the increased effects of these agents in elderly persons and small children.
10. a. Patient teaching measures should include information about potential side effects and potential drug interactions. In addition, safety measures to prevent injury stemming from decreased sensorium must be emphasized.
    b. These medications are most effective when used in conjunction with physical therapy.
11. Tachyphylaxis is the rapid appearance of a progressive decrease in response to a pharmacologically or physiologically active substance after its repetitive administration. Chloral hydrate, an older nonbarbiturate sedative-hypnotic agent, has this characteristic. It is a disadvantage because tachyphylaxis makes the

Copyright © 2002 by Mosby, Inc. All rights reserved.

drug useful for only short-term therapy.

CHAPTER 12
Antiepileptic Agents

Critical Thinking Crossword

Across
  2. Emergency
  6. Primary
 10. Hepatotoxicity
 11. Seizure
 12. Slowly

Down
  1. Secondary
  3. Convulsion
  4. Benzodiazepines
  5. Idiopathic
  6. Phenobarbital
  7. Autoinduction
  8. Epilepsy
  9. Phenytoin

Multiple-choice and short answer

1. d
2. a
3. a
4. c
5. b
6. Carbamazepine undergoes autoinduction, the process whereby a drug increases its own metabolism over time, leading to lower-than-expected drug concentrations.
7. Jeremy's mother should be told that topiramate should be taken whole and not crushed, broken in half, or chewed. It does have a very bitter taste, and seems to be better tolerated with food. She can still give it with the jello, as long as it is whole.

CHAPTER 13
Antiparkinsonian Agents

1. b
2. a
3. c
4. d
5. b
6. a. Dopamine must be given in this form because exogenously administered dopamine cannot pass through the blood-brain barrier; levodopa can.
   b. The addition of carbidopa avoids the high peripheral levels of dopamine and the unwanted side effects induced by the very large doses of levodopa necessary when given alone.
   c. Carbidopa does not cross the blood-brain barrier and thus prevents levodopa breakdown in the periphery. This, in turn, allows levodopa to reach and cross the blood-brain barrier without carbidopa doing so. Once in the brain, the levodopa is then broken down to dopamine, which can be used directly.
7. You must ask whether Mrs. Reynolds is lactating; if so, amantadine is contraindicated.
8. Elderly patients are at risk for urinary retention, especially men with benign prostatic hypertrophy. Jane's neighbor may or may not have the second condition, but his age is a major factor. Jane's age is not a major factor at this time.

CHAPTER 14
Psychotherapeutic Agents

1. m
2. g
3. h
4. o
5. b
6. j
7. k
8. l
9. c
10. n
11. a
12. d
13. i
14. f
15. e
16. c
17. a
18. c
19. b
20. d
21. a. If Carl is taking a benzodiazepine for his anxiety and drinking alcohol, he is probably experiencing benzodiazepine toxicity or overdose.
   b. If ingestion is recent, Carl might be treated with gastric lavage. He might also be given flumazenil to reverse the effect of the benzodiazepine overdose.
22. a. Mr. Delvecchio needs to be aware of the foods and drinks, including red wine, that he can no longer have because they contain tyramine.
   b. It appears that Mr. Delvecchio may have inadvertently ingested something containing tyramine, which has caused a hypertensive crisis.

Copyright © 2002 by Mosby, Inc. All rights reserved.

c. Mr. Delvecchio will probably need to have nifedipine available at all times in the event of tyramine ingestion, which can cause such a sudden and severe reaction.

23. Second-generation antidepressants offer an advantage over other antidepressants because their side/adverse effect profiles are very clean.

CHAPTER 15
Central Nervous System Stimulant Agents

1. b
2. d
3. a
4. c
5. d
6. a. Stacey has narcolepsy.
   b. Methylphenidate, or one of a variety of amphetamines
   c. These agents increase mental alertness, increase motor activity, and diminish the patient's sense of fatigue by stimulating the cerebral cortex and possibly the reticular activating system.
   d. (1) She should take her medication exactly as her physician prescribes, without skipping, omitting, or doubling up on her doses.
      (2) Stacey should avoid other sources of CNS stimulants, in particular caffeine-containing products (e.g., coffee, tea, colas, and chocolate). She should check with her doctor before taking any OTC agent, and she should not consume any substance that contains alcohol.
7. The height and weight of children on methylphenidate should be measured and recorded before therapy is initiated, and their growth rate should be plotted during therapy. The agent's use should be monitored because it may retard growth.

CHAPTER 16
Adrenergic Agents

1. d
2. c
3. d
4. a
5. c
6. a. The alpha-adrenergic activity of this drug causes vasoconstriction in the nasal mucosa. This produces shrinkage of the mucosa and promotes easier nasal breathing.

b. Perhaps she administered the spray too often. Excessive use of nasal decongestants can lead to greater congestion because of a rebound phenomenon.

7. The drug is contraindicated in patients who have a tumor that secretes catecholamines, such as a pheochromocytoma.

8. Dopamine's actions depend on the dose. At low doses, it can dilate blood vessels in the brain, heart, kidneys and mesentery, increasing blood flow to these areas. Increased renal flow may help to remove excess fluid volume. At higher infusion rates, dopamine can improve contractility and cardiac output.

9. Concurrent administration of two adrenergic agents, such as epinephrine and isoproterenol, runs a high risk of precipitating side effects such as tachycardia and hypertension. At least 4 hours should elapse between doses of these medications to prevent serious cardiac dysrhythmias.

CHAPTER 17
Adrenergic-Blocking Agents

1. b
2. a
3. c
4. d
5. d
6. Extravasation can cause vasoconstriction and ultimately tissue death (necrosis). If the vasoconstriction is not reversed quickly, the whole limb can be lost. Phentolamine, an alpha-blocker, can reverse this potent vasoconstriction and restore blood flow to the ischemic, vasoconstricted area. When phentolamine is injected SC in a circular fashion around the extravasation site, it causes alpha-adrenergic receptor blockade and vasodilation. This, in turn, increases blood flow to the ischemic tissue, thus preventing permanent damage.

7. Those that are considered cardioprotective are so because they inhibit stimulation by the circulating catecholamines released during muscle damage, such as that caused by an MI. When a beta-blocker occupies their receptors, the circulating catecholamines cannot bind to their receptors. Thus, the beta-blockers "protect" the heart from being stimulated by these catecholamines, which would only further increase the heart rate and the contractile force, thereby increasing myocardial oxygen demand.

8. She should take her apical pulse for 1 full minute and monitor her blood pressure because of the cardiac depression that can

Copyright © 2002 by Mosby, Inc. All rights reserved.

occur with these agents. In fact, if her systolic blood pressure decreases to less than 100 mm Hg, her pulse decreases to less than 60 beats/min, or her blood pressure continues to decrease, even by a few millimeters of mercury, she should contact her physician. Finally, she should also report any weight gain—especially more than 2 pounds in a week—weakness, shortness of breath, and edema.

CHAPTER 18
Cholinergic Agents

1. h
2. g
3. f
4. b
5. j
6. e
7. i
8. a
9. a
10. b
11. d
12. c
13. b
14. SLUDGE stands for Salivation, Lacrimation, Urinary incontinence, Diarrhea, Gastrointestinal cramps, and Emesis.
15. a. Bethanechol is the drug of choice.
    b. None. Bethanechol is contraindicated in patients with a genitourinary obstruction. The drug should be discontinued immediately.
16. a. Cholinergic crisis.
    b. Tape atropine, the antidote, to the wall next to the patient's bed, or have it available somewhere in Mr. Keegan's room.
17. a. She should experience less eyelid drooping (ptosis), less double vision (diplopia), less difficulty swallowing and chewing, and/or less weakness.
    b. She should report any increased muscle weakness, abdominal cramps, diarrhea, or difficulty breathing.

CHAPTER 19
Cholinergic-Blocking Agents

1. a
2. b
3. d
4. c
5. b
6. Tolterodine (Detrol) is used to treat urinary frequency, urgency, and urge incontinence. Tolterodine appears to have a lower incidence

of dry mouth because of its specificity for the bladder as opposed to the salivary glands. It should be taken with food; the dry mouth that may occur may be best handled by chewing gum, performing frequent mouth care, and keeping hard candy available. The decreased ability to sweat or perspire should be managed by increasing fluids and bulk and avoiding extremes of heat.

7. She can be told to take the larger doses at bedtime because this can help decrease the ulcer pain that is waking her at night.
8. a. Initially, Mr. Miller should be treated with hospitalization, and close, continuous monitoring (including continuous ECG monitoring). The stomach should be emptied through induced emesis with syrup of ipecac if he is awake and nonconvulsive. Fluid therapy and other standard measures used to treat shock should be instituted as needed.
    b. Should he lose consciousness or suffer convulsions, switch to performing lavage instead; use of activated charcoal is effective in removing a drug that is already absorbed.
    c. In the case of hallucinations, physostigmine has proved helpful, although its use is somewhat controversial because of severe adverse effects with routine use.
9. Antihistamines can have additive effects on cholinergic blockers, resulting in increased effects.

CHAPTER 20
Positive Inotropic Agents

1. b
2. c
3. d
4. a
5. b
6. Vomiting, headache, fatigue, and dysrhythmia are adverse effects of cardiac glycosides. A serum potassium level of greater than 5 mEq/L indicates digoxin toxicity. Mrs. Chin may require Digibind for digoxin overdose.
7. Because of digoxin's fairly long duration of action and half-life, the physician has prescribed a loading, or "digitalizing," dose for Mr. Davis to bring the serum levels of the drug up to a therapeutic level more quickly. The usual loading dose is 1 to 1.5 mg/day, whereas the usual maintenance dose is 0.125 to 0.5 mg/day.
8. The therapeutic window is the range of the drug level in the blood that is considered therapeutic. Because digoxin has such a narrow therapeutic

Copyright © 2002 by Mosby, Inc. All rights reserved.

window, patients require constant monitoring for side/adverse effects and toxic symptoms.

9. Increased urinary output and decreased dyspnea and fatigue are therapeutic effects of digoxin. The constipation needs to be assessed. Mr. Ferris should not be allowed to consume large amounts of bran or other foods high in fiber because the bran will bind to the digitalis and make less of the drug available for absorption.

10. a. Amrinone increases the force of contraction (inotropic effect) and relaxes the blood vessels (lusitropic effect), causing a reduction in afterload, or the force that the heart has to pump against to eject its volume.

   b. Phosphodiesterase inhibitors do not require a receptor-mediated effect to increase contraction, and increased dosages are not needed to maintain positive results; therefore unwanted cardiac side effects do not occur.

   c. Thrombocytopenia.

CHAPTER 21
Antidysrhythmic Agents

1. d
2. c
3. b
4. c
5. a
6. a. Class II antidysrhythmics, or beta-blockers, are indicated because they have been shown to significantly reduce the incidence of sudden cardiac death after MI.

   b. If Mr. Killian had asthma, most of the class II drugs would be contraindicated.

   c. Myasthenia gravis is not a contraindication to class II drugs.

7. Amiodarone is considered a drug of last resort. Although it is very effective, amiodarone can penetrate and concentrate in the adipose tissue of any organ in the body, where it may cause unwanted effects. It may cause either hypothyroidism or hyperthyroidism, corneal microdeposits, pulmonary toxicity, and even dysrhythmias. Amiodarone has a very long half-life, and the side effects may take months to subside.

8. a. The verapamil Ms. Lionel is taking is effective in treating her hypertension. Also, drugs that interact with verapamil include antihypertensive agents, which enhance the risk of hypotension and heart failure.

   b. The physician may prescribe adenosine, which is useful for the treatment of PSVT that has failed to respond to verapamil.

9. Lidocaine must be injected IM or IV; when lidocaine is taken orally, the liver metabolizes most of it to inactive metabolites. However, Mr. Maxwell is exhibiting some adverse reactions to the lidocaine, and the physician should be notified.

10. Mrs. Inez should be told to not double up on her medication. The physician should be contacted about the missed dose and about Mrs. Inez's symptoms of chest pain and dizziness, which are adverse effects of the quinidine.

CHAPTER 22
Antianginal Agents

1. c
2. c
3. b
4. d
5. a
6. Call 911 and assist the patient until the ambulance arrives. At this time you don't know the man's condition, and you certainly can't administer someone else's medication to him. Even if you could, you know that Peritrate is recommended only for long-term prophylactic treatment of angina—not acute treatment—and that it is not a sublingual form of nitroglycerin anyway. Isordil is available in a sublingual form, but again, you can't administer another person's medication, especially to someone with an undetermined condition.

7. Ms. Vickers might be taking a beta-blocker. Fatigue and lethargy are the most common patient complaints with the use of beta-blockers, and mental depression can be exacerbated, particularly in the elderly. Also, one of the CNS adverse effects of beta-blockers is the occurrence of unusual dreams.

8. Theresa should always include in her journal a description of the activity she was performing at the time her angina occurred. Also, she must keep the tablets in an airtight, dark glass bottle away from sunlight, because the active ingredient in nitroglycerin is easily destroyed.

CHAPTER 23
Antihypertensive Agents

Critical Thinking Crossword

Across
1. Secondary
5. Idiopathic
7. Orthostatic
8. Vasodilators

Copyright © 2002 by Mosby, Inc. All rights reserved.

Down
  2. Essential
  3. Primary
  4. Diuretics
  6. Ace

Multiple-choice and short answer

  1. c
  2. c
  3. b
  4. a
  5. d
  6. The newer drugs produce fewer side effects and have more selective actions.
  7. a. Other hypotensive agents should be administered as soon as the blood pressure is under control. Start the drug at an initial rate of 0.5 to 1.0 mg/min, with subsequent gradual increases in the rate until the desired blood pressure response is achieved. Average infusion rates range between 1 to 4 mg/min and are generally titrated to maintain a systolic blood pressure of between 100 and 120 mm Hg.
     b. Tachyphylaxis develops in 24 to 72 hours.
  8. a. Captopril is probably best for Irene. In critically ill patients, a drug with a short half-life, such as captopril, is better because if problems arise, they will be short-lived. Also, Irene has liver dysfunction, so captopril has an advantage in that it is not a prodrug (a prodrug is inactive in its present form and must be biotransformed in the liver to its active form to be effective).
     b. Because of his history of poor compliance, Kory would benefit from a drug with a long half-life and duration of action, which he would need to take only once a day. In that case, one of the newer ACE inhibitors—benazepril, fosinopril, lisinopril, quinapril, or ramipril—would be best.
  9. There is a first-dose effect with prazosin. This means that the patient will experience a considerable drop in blood pressure after taking the first dose, so he should take it while lying down or before bedtime and arise slowly. This first-dose effect decreases with time or with a reduction in the dose, as ordered by the physician.

CHAPTER 24
Diuretic Agents

  1. c
  2. e
  3. d
  4. g
  5. f
  6. h
  7. b
  8. a
  9. b
 10. c
 11. a
 12. d
 13. c
 14. a. Ms. Andersen was probably prescribed a carbonic anhydrase inhibitor (CAI).
     b. An undesirable effect of the CAIs is that they elevate the blood glucose level, causing glycosuria in diabetic patients.
 15. a. In order for mannitol to be effective in treating ARF, enough renal blood flow and glomerular filtration must exist to enable the drug to reach the tubules.
     b. Mannitol is always administered IV through a filter because it can crystallize when exposed to low temperatures (which is more likely to occur when concentrations exceed 15%).
     c. Arthur's headache and chills are probably side effects of the mannitol therapy. At this time, the therapy should be continued, but Arthur should be monitored for the development of more serious adverse effects.
 16. a. Mr. Ferrara will be prescribed spironolactone in high doses; this drug is used often for the treatment of ascites associated with cirrhosis of the liver.
     b. His serum potassium level will need to be monitored frequently because he has impaired renal function.
 17. a. Impotence and decreased libido are among the side effects of thiazide; Brendan is possibly experiencing these effects.
     b. He should stop eating licorice because its consumption can lead to an additive hypokalemia in patients taking thiazide. Brendan's fatigue may be the result of drug toxicity and should be evaluated.
 18. It is likely that Mrs. Hill's neighbor was prescribed one of the potassium-sparing diuretics and thus was not instructed to eat additional potassium-rich foods. Mrs. Hill should follow the dietary recommendations provided for her, not for her neighbor.

Copyright © 2002 by Mosby, Inc. All rights reserved.

19. a. Patients should keep a log of their daily weights to monitor for changes in fluid volume.
    b. A weight gain of 2 or more pounds a day or 5 or more pounds a week should be reported.
    c. Vomiting and/or diarrhea can precipitate electrolyte and fluid loss.

CHAPTER 25
Fluids and Electrolytes

1. d
2. d
3. a
4. c
5. b
6. Albumin contains particles that are all the same size; the other colloids contain a combination of both small and large particles. While the other colloids are metabolized in the liver and excreted by the kidneys, albumin is metabolized by the reticuloendothelial system and excreted by the kidneys and intestines.
7. a. Blood products.
   b. They are the only fluids that contain hemoglobin.
   c. They are natural products that require human donors, which means that they can be incompatible with a recipient's immune system; these products can also transmit pathogens from the donor to the recipient.
8. a. Tanya is exhibiting early symptoms of hypokalemia.
   b. She should eat foods high in potassium, such as bananas, orange juice, and apricots.
9. a. Hyponatremia.
   b. Mr. Sanchez can take in sodium by eating foods high in salt, such as catsup, mustard, cured meats, and potato chips.
   c. Vomiting is a symptom of hyponatremia, as well as a side effect of oral administration of sodium chloride.
10. a. Victor's general appearance and affect.
    b. Although it is possible for pathogens such as AIDS to be transmitted via blood products, Victor's wife should be reassured that techniques are now used that have drastically reduced the incidence of such problems.
    c. Every 15 minutes or more often if needed.
    d. Victor's restlessness and increased pulse need to be reported to the physician immediately because these are signs of a reaction to the blood product, and the transfusion should be stopped immediately.

CHAPTER 26
Coagulation Modifier Agents

1. j
2. m
3. i
4. k
5. l
6. b
7. a
8. h
9. g
10. d
11. f
12. b
13. b
14. a
15. c
16. a
17. a. Yes! The injection site should not be massaged or rubbed before or after the injection.
    b. The APTT (activated partial thromboplastin time) is the test most commonly used.
18. a. The anticoagulant effects of heparin can be reversed with protamine sulfate.
    b. In general, for every 100 units of heparin, 1 mg of protamine can reverse the effects.
19. In the event that the warfarin therapy must be reinstated, resistance to its effect will be encountered because a large dose of vitamin K will maintain its reversal effects for up to a week.
20. a. The antifibrinolytics (specifically, aminocaproic acid) are used to stop excessive oozing from surgical sites, such as chest tubes; they are also successful in reducing the total blood loss and duration of bleeding in the postoperative period.
    b. Via IV infusion, 4 to 5 gm during the first hour, then 1 to 1.25 gm at 1-hour intervals up to a daily maximum of 30 g.
21. Desmopressin is used in patients with type I von Willebrand's disease; it increases the levels of clotting factor VIII.
22. a. No. Alteplase is present in our bodies in a natural state, so it does not induce an antigen-antibody reaction.
    b. The Activase can be readministered because it has a very short half-life of 5 minutes.
23. a. They are possible indications of bleeding problems related to the anticoagulation therapy.
    b. Ursula might also be exhibiting a change in pulse rate or rhythm, blood pressure, or level of consciousness.
    c. Notify the physician immediately.

Copyright © 2002 by Mosby, Inc. All rights reserved.

CHAPTER 27
Antilipemic Agents

1. d
2. b
3. a
4. b
5. c
6. a. Fibric acid derivative—it is believed that these agents work by activating lipoprotein lipase, an enzyme responsible for the breakdown of cholesterol.
   b. Lipid-lowering agent and vitamin—exact mechanism unknown; beneficial effects are believed to be related to its ability to inhibit lipolysis in adipose tissue, decrease esterification of triglycerides in the liver, and increase the activity of lipoprotein lipase.
   c. HMG-CoA reductase inhibitor—reduces blood cholesterol by decreasing the rate of cholesterol production.
   d. Bile acid sequestrant—lowers plasma LDL by enhancing the efficiency of the receptor-mediated removal of LDL from plasma. The result of ion-exchange resin binding to bile acids is an insoluble resin-bile complex that is excreted by means of the feces.
7. Unless Mr. Harris has additional risk factors, his high LDL level alone does not warrant drug therapy at this time. All reasonable non-pharmaceutical means of controlling Mr. Harris' LDL level need to be tried and found to fail before he is given drug therapy. Mr. Harris needs to find time in his busy schedule to exercise and eat more wisely.
8. Mr. Jahnke's age and smoking are risk factors, as is the fact that his father died suddenly of heart disease before the age of 55. Mr. Jahnke's asthma and arthritis are not risk factors, nor is his blood pressure. Mr. Jahnke's HDL is above 60 mg/dl, so it is considered a negative risk factor and can be subtracted from the total number of positive risk factors.
9. Mrs. Kim is experiencing constipation and belching associated with cholestyramine use (she may also be experiencing heartburn, nausea, and bloating). Mrs. Kim requires extra patient teaching and support to help her maintain compliance with the drug therapy; she should be assured that these adverse effects will probably diminish over time.
10. No! Justus is not a candidate for niacin therapy for two reasons: (1) niacin is not recommended with lovastatin because it can lead to the development of rhabdomyolysis, and (2) niacin is contraindicated in patients with peptic ulcer.
11. First, it is imperative that Mrs. Nguyen take her antihypertensive and Questran at different times of the day because pronounced drug interactions can result when the bile acid sequestrants and other drugs are taken concurrently. All other drugs should be taken at least 1 hour before or 4 to 6 hours after the administration of antilipemics. Also, the powder form of Questran should be allowed to dissolve slowly in at least 2 ounces of fluid, without stirring, for at least 1 minute—stirring causes the powder to clump. The powder may not mix totally in the glass, and more fluid may need to be added to the glass. The powder may also be mixed thoroughly with food, or fruit, such as crushed pineapple.

CHAPTER 28
Pituitary Agents

1. a. glucocorticoids, mineralocorticoids, androgen
   b. Corticotropin
   c. Regulates anabolic processes related to growth and adaptation to stressors; promotes skeletal and muscle growth; increases protein synthesis; increases liver glycogenolysis; increases fat mobilization
   d. Somatropin
   e. Antidiuretic hormone
   f. Vasopressin, lypressin, and desmopressin
2. c
3. d
4. b
5. d
6. a
7. a. Alexis might very well benefit from administration of corticotropin not only to treat the pain associated with inflammation, but also to produce increased comfort and muscle strength.
   b. Cautions include checking to see whether Alexis may be pregnant or nursing. Also, does she have liver disease, mental illness, gout, hypothyroidism, or latent TB? Drug interactions you should be mindful of may occur with alcohol, aspirin, steroids, diuretics, and amphotericin B. Contraindications include, of course, an allergy to the drug. In addition, do not give this drug in the presence of osteoporosis, CHF, ulcer disease, scleroderma, fungal infections, recent surgery, or primary adrenocortical dysfunction.
   c. Other assessment parameters include obtaining baseline vital signs, electrolyte values, blood glucose levels, chest x-ray,

Copyright © 2002 by Mosby, Inc. All rights reserved.

CBC, intake and output, daily weight, and cortisol levels. It is important to assess for allergy to pork because of cross-sensitivity.

d. Patient teaching plans should include issues listed at length in the "Patient Teaching Tips" box in this chapter.

8. In addition to information about proper subcutaneous injection techniques, the teaching plan should include a reminder of the dosage form and amount and the importance of compliance with therapy. Warn Patricia's parents not to administer a discolored or cloudy solution but to return it to the clinic. Finally, show them how to keep a journal of Patricia's growth measurements.

9. a. Mr. Collins will probably be found to have diabetes insipidus; if so, he will benefit from treatment with vasopressin or lypressin.

b. Assessment strategies should include evaluating pulse, vital signs, intake and output, daily weight, and edema. Note that treatment should proceed only with great caution if Mr. Collins has coronary artery disease. However, in the face of chronic renal disease or an allergy to the drug, Mr. Collins will be ineligible for this treatment.

c. Treatment will be via nasal spray 1 to 2 sprays administered 1 to 2 times in each nostril QID. This should increase water resorption in the distal tubules and collecting ducts of the nephron, performing all the physiologic functions of ADH.

d. It should eliminate his severe thirst and decrease his urinary output.

e. Any teaching plan should include encouraging Mr. Collins to carry his medication with him at all times. He should use the nasal spray according to the instructions and only after he has cleared his nasal passages. The spray should not be inhaled. Common side/adverse effects that could apply to Mr. Collins include drowsiness, headache, lethargy, flushing, nausea, heartburn, cramps, increased blood pressure, nasal irritation and congestion, tremor, sweating, and vertigo.

CHAPTER 29
Thyroid and Antithyroid Agents

Critical Thinking Crossword

Across
  3. Secondary
  6. Thyroxine
  7. Primary

Down
  1. Levothyroxine
  2. Hyperthyroidism
  4. Propylthiouracil
  5. Tertiary
  6. Thyrotropin

Multiple-choice and short answer

1. d
2. d
3. a
4. b
5. c
6. Mrs. Westin probably has hypothyroidism, which may result in the formation of a goiter, an enlargement of the thyroid gland resulting from its overstimulation by elevated levels of TSH. She may benefit from one of the thyroid agents, including thyroid, thyroglobulin, levothyroxine, liothyronine, or liotrix. Levothyroxine is generally preferred because—since it is chemically pure at 100% T_4—its hormonal content is standardized; therefore its effect is predictable.

7. Even if we can determine that those last several symptoms are due to menopause, the combination of the rest of the symptoms, plus her history, indicate the strong possibility that Ms. Hilton has hyperthyroidism. This is especially worth investigating since it is sometimes caused by Graves' disease.

8. In some types of hyperthyroidism, such as that seen in Graves' disease, long-term administration may induce a spontaneous remission. However, most patients eventually require surgery or radioactive iodine therapy to ablate the condition.

CHAPTER 30
Antidiabetic and Hypoglycemic Agents

1. b
2. d
3. a
4. c
5. a

Copyright © 2002 by Mosby, Inc. All rights reserved.

6. b
7. Site rotation of insulin injections should be within the same location for about 1 week, but at least 1/2 to 1 inch away from the previous site. For example, areas within the right arm the first week, then within the left thigh the next week, etc. Some practitioners recommend only using the abdomen because of more complete absorption.
8. a. Alice's diet should include a high intake of protein and a low intake of carbohydrates.
   b. The brain needs a constant amount of glucose to function; thus the central nervous system manifestations of hypoglycemia (such as irritability) are often the first to appear.
   c. In the conscious person, use glucagons, glucose tablets or gel, corn syrup, honey, fruit juice, or a non-diet soft drink, or a small snack such as crackers or half a sandwich.
9. a. Bill should check the order at least three times and have another registered nurse check the prepared injection to be sure it is in accordance with the physician's order.
   b. You, of course! Novolin-R is regular insulin, and regular insulin is the only insulin that is clear.
   c. If left at room temperature, the insulin in the vial should have been used within 1 month; otherwise, it should have been refrigerated.
10. a. Alec requires an intermediate-acting insulin.
    b. Alec's religious beliefs might prohibit him from using insulin made from pork.
11. a. Mrs. Franklin needs to make some significant lifestyle changes. She must stop smoking, lose weight, and exercise regularly, which will help with both the high blood glucose level and the hypertension.
    b. Mrs. Franklin should continue with her exercise and weight loss program; however, because her blood glucose level is still elevated, she also requires an oral antidiabetic agent.
12. a. Hypoglycemia.
    b. Dennis may have been drinking alcohol. The hypoglycemic effect of sulfonylurea agents is increased when they are taken with alcohol, and Dennis's symptoms of profound flushing of the skin and face are indicative of the "chlorpropamide-alcohol flush." It is most prominent with chlorpropamide (Diabinese) use.

13. a. The second-generation sulfonylureas have many advantages over the older agents, including much greater potency. Also, chlorpropamide is dependent on the kidneys for elimination and can cause toxicity in patients with decreased renal function.
    b. Glipizide is indicated; glyburide is less desirable for the treatment of short-term elevations in blood glucose level because of its relatively slow onset of action.
    c. Mr. Dressel should contact his physician immediately. He may require a change in his diabetic treatment while he is sick because vomiting and inability to eat can cause a change in his blood glucose levels.

CHAPTER 31
Adrenal Agents

1. a
2. c
3. d
4. b
5. c
6. Ms. Rivera's glucocorticoid can interact with aspirin and other NSAIDs, producing additive effects. Also, she should avoid persons with infections because her own immune system is suppressed.
7. a. The use of systemic glucocorticoids with antidiabetic agents may reduce the hypoglycemic effect of those agents. A baseline blood glucose level should be determined, and Peter should be monitored for any problems.
   b. Oral systemic adrenal agents should be taken with food or milk.
8. Intervene! The student nurse should, while wearing gloves, apply the medication with a sterile tongue depressor or cotton-tipped applicator—if the skin is intact. If the skin is not intact, a sterile technique should be used.
9. In addition to routine teaching about inhaler administration technique, Nina should be instructed to clean out the oral cavity with mouthwash to prevent an oral fungal infection from developing.

CHAPTER 32
Women's Health Agents

1. d
2. c
3. a
4. b
5. b

Copyright © 2002 by Mosby, Inc. All rights reserved.

6. a. Ask Isabelle if she is taking medication for her depression. Estrogen therapy is indicated for the symptoms of menopause, but the use of estrogen with a tricyclic antidepressant may result in a toxic response.
   b. The smallest dose of estrogen that alleviates the symptoms is used for the shortest possible time.
7. a. The physician will probably prescribe medroxyprogesterone, which is indicated for treatment of secondary amenorrhea.
   b. Ms. Keller's dose of antidiabetic agent may need to be adjusted because of a possible decrease in glucose tolerance when progestins and antidiabetic agents are taken together.
8. a. Maybe Jacklyn's prescription could be switched to a 28-day form of Ortho-Novum, which is taken for all 28 days of the menstrual cycle, rather than 3 weeks on and 1 week off.
   b. One of the benefits of oral contraceptives is decreased blood loss during menstruation.
9. a. The physician will probably prescribe terbutaline or ritodrine. These agents work by stimulating the beta-adrenergic receptors located on the uterine smooth muscle. The muscle then relaxes and stops contracting.
   b. Ms. O'Hara is placed in the left lateral recumbent position in order to minimize hypotension and increase renal blood flow.
   c. Hyperglycemia and hypokalemia are metabolic adverse effects of tocolytic therapy.
10. a. Gonadotropin and menotropins are customarily used together. The Pergonal is given to stimulate ovarian follicular growth and maturation. Then, a single, large dose of gonadotropin is given to induce ovulation.
    b. The 9 to 12 days of FSH/LH gonadotropins (Pergonal) injections and then a single dose of chorionic gonadotropin (hCG) may be repeated a second and third time if needed.
11. Mrs. Ingalls needs to know that smoking can diminish the therapeutic effects of the estrogen she's taking. Also, she should be cautioned to wear sunscreen while in Aruba, because estrogen makes the skin more susceptible to sunburn.
12. a. Mrs. Simmons is assuming that the medication is estrogen therapy. Alendronate (Fosamax) is indicated to prevent osteoporosis in postmenopausal women. You will need to explain to her that it is the first nonestrogen, nonhormonal medication used for prevention of bone loss in the early postmenopausal period, and for women who experience early menopause, the dose of 5 mg daily is recommended.
    b. We know that she experienced early menopause; other risk factors associated with the development of postmenopausal osteoporosis include thin body build, Caucasian or Asian race, family history of osteoporosis, and moderately low bone mass. She would need to be assessed for these other risk factors.

CHAPTER 33
Men's Health Agents

1. b
2. d
3. a
4. c
5. c
6. IM testosterone is given deep in the upper outer quadrant of the gluteus muscle injection site.
7. a. Testosterone's poor performance in oral dose form is due to the fact that most of a dose is metabolized and destroyed by the liver before it can reach the circulation.
   b. Methyltestosterone and fluoxymesterone are both testosterone derivatives that are effective when given buccally or orally. With either drug, contraindications that could apply to Mr. Michaels include significant cardiac, hepatic or renal dysfunction, breast carcinoma, or known or suspected prostate cancer.
8. a. No. The manufacturer's guidelines suggest that the patient not swallow, chew, or eat the buccal tablet but that it be completely absorbed.
   b. Patients taking any hormone-related agent should never abruptly stop.
9. a. Finasteride works by inhibiting the enzymatic process responsible for converting testosterone to 5-alpha-dihydrotestosterone (DHT), which is the principal androgen responsible for stimulating prostatic growth. It can dramatically lower the prostatic DHT concentrations, thereby reducing the testosterone concentrations and causing the hypertrophied prostate to decrease in size.
   b. Patient teaching plans should include rationales for therapy and a full disclosure of side effects.

Copyright © 2002 by Mosby, Inc. All rights reserved.

10. In addition to more general information, a patient teaching plan for the patient taking danazol should include the following: it should be taken with food or milk to minimize the gastric upset often associated with its use. In addition, Mrs. Thiele should report any abnormal vaginal discharge or bleeding and should perform routine breast examinations.
11. a. Sildenafil (Viagra) should be used cautiously in patients with renal disorders, hypertension, diabetes, and cardiovascular disease, especially if they are taking nitrates due to enhanced postural hypotensive effects and potential syncope.
    b. Headache, UTI, diarrhea, rash, dizziness, flushing and dyspepsia are the most common adverse effects reported. In addition, Viagra is highly protein-bound and may interact with many drugs. Mr. A. should check with the doctor before taking any other medication.

CHAPTER 34
Antihistamines, Decongestants, Antitussives, and Expectorants

1. d
2. a
3. b
4. c
5. b
6. The antihistamines cannot push off histamine that is already bound to its receptor. Because they compete with histamine for unoccupied receptors, they work best when given early in a reaction, before all of the histamine binds to receptors.
7. Yes. The traditional antihistamines have anticholinergic effects, which may make them more effective in some cases. Patients respond to and tolerate these agents quite well. Also, because many traditional antihistamines are generically available, they are much less expensive.
8. a. James's diabetes should not affect his treatment.
    b. The topical diphenhydramine might come in combination with an agent such as calamine, camphor, or zinc oxide.
    c. Diphenhydramine has the greatest range of therapeutic indications of any of the available antihistamines. It is used for the relief or prevention of histamine-mediated allergies, motion sickness, the treatment of Parkinson's disease, as a sleep aid, and—in conjunction with epinephrine—in the management of anaphylaxis.

9. No! Mrs. Ling is likely experiencing rebound congestion caused by sustained use of the naphazoline for several days.
10. Keith is exhibiting symptoms of the cardiovascular effects that can occur when a topically applied adrenergic nasal decongestant is somewhat absorbed into the bloodstream.
11. Benzonatate's mechanism of action is entirely different from that of the other agents. It suppresses the cough reflex by numbing the stretch receptors, thus keeping the cough reflex from being stimulated in the medulla. It has fewer drug interactions than the narcotic antitussives and dextromethorphan.
12. Ask Irene whether she is taking any thyroid medication. A drug interaction (an additive hypothyroid effect) can occur if she takes an expectorant with an antithyroid agent. Irene should call her physician before she goes to the drugstore.
13. First, Lisa's brother received Robitussin A-C, a narcotic antitussive containing codeine, for his cough. Lisa has been prescribed Robitussin, an expectorant, for her nonproductive cough associated with bronchitis. Second, even if the two children were prescribed the same drug, Lisa is only 5 years old and requires a smaller dosage than her brother.

CHAPTER 35
Bronchodilators and Other Respiratory Agents

1. a
2. d
3. d
4. b
5. c
6. The cause of idiopathic (or intrinsic) asthma is unknown; allergic asthma is caused by hypersensitivity to an allergen in the environment. Idiopathic asthma is not mediated by IgE; allergic asthma is.
7. Intravenous aminophylline is used in patients with status asthmaticus but usually after a fast-acting beta-agonist (like epinephrine) has been tried. In Ms. Ward's case this approach is not possible. Beta-agonists are contraindicated in patients with convulsive disorders.
8. Theophylline and the other xanthine derivatives are used as adjunctive therapy for the relief of pulmonary edema and paroxysmal nocturnal dyspnea in patients with left-sided heart failure. These medications increase the force of contraction in a failing heart and dilate the airways.
9. Tom is exhibiting some side effects of theophylline therapy, and the level in his blood is

Copyright © 2002 by Mosby, Inc. All rights reserved.

probably too high (the common therapeutic range for theophylline in the blood is 10 to 20 mg/dl). Tom may require a reduction in dosage.

10. You need to know how much Willie weighs. The pediatric dosage of epinephrine SC is 10 μg/kg/dose.

11. Sylvia is exhibiting dose-related adverse effects of the albuterol, probably caused by using it too frequently. Sylvia needs to be reminded to use her medication exactly as prescribed.

12. a. Anticholinergics, corticosteroids, and indirect-acting agents.
    b. Of concern is Mrs. Voss's glaucoma. Ipratropium bromide (an anticholinergic) is contraindicated in patients with glaucoma, and corticosteroids should be used with caution in patients with glaucoma.

13. a. The disadvantage to administering the corticosteroids orally is that they can then have systemic effects, such as adrenocortical insufficiency, increased susceptibility to infection, fluid and electrolyte disturbances, endocrine effects, dermatologic effects, and nervous system effects. They can also interact with other systemically administered drugs. (The advantage to administering corticosteroids by inhalation is that their action is limited to the topical site of action—the lungs. In that way they have no systemic effects and cannot interact with other systemically administered drugs.)
    b. Yes. The use of an inhaled corticosteroid frequently allows for a reduction in the daily dose of the systemic corticosteroid.

14. a. Indirect-acting antiasthmatic agents, such as cromolyn, are recommended for the prevention of exercise-induced bronchospasm and bronchospasm induced by exposure to factors such as cold dry air, environmental pollutants, and allergens. Cromolyn is most popularly administered by a nebulizer.
    b. During treatment, Mr. Wells might experience bronchospasms. If bronchospasms continue, his condition should be stabilized, the session discontinued, and the physician notified.
    c. Mr. Wells should be told that the cromolyn must be administered consistently and that the therapeutic effects may take up to 4 weeks to occur. He should also understand how to administer the medication and be told to gargle and rinse his mouth with water afterward to minimize irritation to

the throat and oral mucosa. He should also avoid precipitating factors when possible.

15. a. The CNS-stimulating effects of the xanthines may be enhanced in children.
    b. It depends. Theophylline tablets come in regular and extended-release forms. The extended-release form, of course, cannot be crushed.

16. Ms. Weaver is in need of additional patient education regarding her corticosteroid treatment! Her oral contraceptive, along with several other agents, can interact with the corticosteroids. Also, the physician should be informed of her weight gain in the event that it is an effect of the corticosteroid and not the result of holiday overeating. (Any weight gain of more than 5 pounds per week should be reported by the patient taking a corticosteroid.) There are several other issues you may want to review with Ms. Weaver: abruptly discontinuing the medication can lead to serious consequences; she should wear an ID bracelet identifying her as a steroid user; and she should report any cushingoid symptoms immediately.

CHAPTER 36
Antibiotics

Critical Thinking Crossword

Across
1. Bacteriostatic
3. Cephalosporin
8. Macrolide
9. Tetracycline

Down
1. Bactericidal
2. Superinfection
4. Prophylactic
5. Aminoglycoside
6. Sulfonamide
7. Penicillin

Multiple-choice and short answer

1. d
2. d
3. a
4. b
5. c
6. c
7. Cefoxitin (Mefoxin) is frequently used in patients undergoing abdominal or colorectal surgeries because it can kill the bacteria that usually reside in these areas.

Copyright © 2002 by Mosby, Inc. All rights reserved.

8. a. Sean should not take the doxycycline with milk because that can result in a significant reduction in the oral absorption of the drug. Sean should also be aware that tetracyclines can cause photosensitivity—he should stay out of the sun.

   b. The diarrhea is probably the result of alteration of the intestinal flora caused by the drug therapy.

9. a. Ototoxicity and nephrotoxicity. Ototoxicity's symptoms include dizziness, tinnitus, and hearing loss; nephrotoxicity's symptoms include urinary casts, proteinuria, and increased BUN and serum creatinine levels. Keeping the drug blood levels (peak and trough) within a certain therapeutic range can help to prevent those toxicities.

   b. The aminoglycosides and penicillins are often used together because they have a synergistic effect; that is, the combined effect of the two agents is greater than that of either agent alone.

CHAPTER 37
Antiviral Agents

1. d
2. b
3. a
4. c
5. b
6. Any drug that kills a virus can also kill healthy cells. There are few agents that can kill only the virus and not harm the body's cells. Viruses are difficult to kill because often by the time they are discovered, they have finished replicating. At that point, it is too late for antiviral agents, which interfere with viral replication, to work.
7. Yes. Zidovudine, the only anti-HIV agent known to prolong patient survival, can be used for maternal/fetal treatment. After 14 weeks of pregnancy, Amy can receive an oral agent. During labor she can receive the agent IV. Drug therapy for the infant can begin within 12 hours of delivery and continue for 6 weeks.
8. a. Acyclovir (Zovirax) is indicated for the varicella-zoster virus (shingles).

   b. Bailey's daily fluid intake should be at least 2400 ml while she is taking the acyclovir. Also, acyclovir capsules may be taken with food.

   c. Bailey will be treated with acyclovir again; it is the drug of choice for treatment of both initial and recurrent episodes of shingles.

9. a. Cary should use a glove when applying the topical Zovirax to the affected area, which should be kept clean and dry. Also, he should not use any other creams or ointments on the area.

   b. Cary's herpes cannot be "cured," although the Zovirax will help to manage the symptoms.

   c. Stress the importance of treatment for Cary and his sexual partners, and discuss with him how to prevent transmission of the virus.

10. a. Ribavirin is used to treat infections caused by RSV.

    b. Yes. Brenda's treatment will last at least 3 days but not more than 7 days.

11. a. Nurses should wash their hands before and after administering the medication to prevent contamination of the site and the spread of the infection. They must also adhere to the Standard Precautions.

    b. Side/adverse effects of trifluridine include burning, swelling, stinging, photophobia, and pain.

    c. Trifluridine is applied only topically because significant liver and bone marrow toxicities can occur if the drug is given orally.

12. a. The patient may be experiencing zidovudine's major dose-limiting adverse effect, which is bone marrow suppression.

    b. Eduardo should mix the powder solution in at least 4 ounces of water—not fruit juice or juice containing acid—and drink it immediately. It should be taken on an empty stomach 1 hour before meals, or 2 hours after meals.

    c. No. Antacids taken concurrently with didanosine can cause increased absorption of the didanosine, which is a positive effect.

13. No. Your co-worker is doing fine. Acyclovir administered by IV infusion is first diluted in sterile water or in a solution recommended by the manufacturer and is administered slowly over at least 1 hour.

CHAPTER 38
Antitubercular Agents

1. a
2. b
3. d
4. c
5. a
6. a. Liver function studies should be performed because of the hepatic impairment

Copyright © 2002 by Mosby, Inc. All rights reserved.

INH can cause. CBC, Hgb level, and Hct value should be checked because of the hematologic disorders INH can cause.

   b. It is possible that Diane is a slow acetylator. Acetylation, the process by which INH is metabolized in the liver, requires certain enzymes to break down the INH. In slow acetylators who have a genetic deficiency of the enzymes, the INH accumulates. The dosage of INH may need to be adjusted downward in these patients.

7. a. Streptomycin is administered intramuscularly, deep in a large muscle mass, and the sites are rotated.

   b. The side/adverse effects of streptomycin are ototoxicity, nephrotoxicity, and blood dyscrasia.

   c. Although it may not be a concern in terms of Ms. Innes's streptomycin therapy, oral contraceptives become ineffective when given with rifampin. If rifampin is part of her therapy, Ms. Innes should switch to another form of birth control.

8. A thorough eye examination may be called for before the institution of therapy, because ethambutol can cause a decrease in visual acuity resulting from optic neuritis. Contraindications to the use of INH and ethambutol include optic neuritis.

9. a. George's gout is a consideration; pyrazinamide can cause hyperuricemia, so gout or flare-ups of gout can occur in susceptible patients. His diabetes is a concern too; ethambutol should be used cautiously in patients with diabetes. Finally, streptomycin should be used very carefully in the elderly.

   b. George should monitor his blood glucose levels using a glucometer because INH can cause hyperglycemia.

10. a. Mr. Fiore needs to know that his compliance with therapy is essential for achieving a cure. Although he is keeping his follow-up appointments, Mr. Fiore also needs to take his medication as ordered. He should be warned to not consume alcohol, and he should be encouraged to take care of himself with adequate nutrition, rest, and relaxation.

   b. The therapeutic response can be confirmed by results of laboratory studies (culture and sensitivity tests) and chest x-ray findings.

11. a. Frannie, like all patients taking antitubercular agents, needs to be compliant with the therapy and keep her follow-up appointments. She should be reminded that she is contagious (during the initial period of the illness); she should wash her hands frequently, and cover her mouth when coughing or sneezing. Frannie also needs adequate nutrition and rest.

   b. It is likely that Frannie is on rifampin therapy. She should be told that her urine, stool, saliva, sputum, sweat, or tears may become reddish orange and that this is an effect of rifampin therapy.

CHAPTER 39
Antifungal Agents

1. j
2. e
3. f
4. g
5. a
6. c
7. h
8. i
9. d
10. b
11. c
12. b
13. d
14. b
15. a
16. Mycotic infections are very difficult to kill, and research into new agents has occurred at a slow pace—in part, because the chemical concentrations of the experimental agents cannot be tolerated by humans.
17. a. Fluconazole (Diflucan) can pass into the CSF (unlike itraconazole), making it effective in the treatment of cryptococcal meningitis. It is considered to be the most effective of the imidazoles for treating several infections.

   b. Unfortunately, Mr. Kim will need to remain on the medication (at a reduced dosage) for 10 to 12 weeks after his negative CSF culture.

18. a. The amphotericin B should be diluted according to the manufacturer's guidelines.

   b. Fever, chills, hypotension, tachycardia, malaise, muscle and joint pain, anorexia, nausea and vomiting, and headache.

   c. No. Almost all patients experience these effects. To decrease their severity, pretreatment with an antipyretic, antihistamines, and antiemetics may be given.

19. Lewis should be aware that he will be taking the medication for 2 to 6 weeks, until the infection clears. During that time, he should

Copyright © 2002 by Mosby, Inc. All rights reserved.

avoid alcohol because of the Antabuse-type reaction that could occur, and he should take the medication with food to avoid GI upset. Griseofulvin also causes photosensitivity, so Lewis should avoid the sun or use sunscreen.

CHAPTER 40
Antimalarial, Antiprotozoal, and Anthelmintic Agents

1. a
2. b
3. c
4. b
5. b
6. Malaria is caused by *Plasmodium* organisms. During the asexual stage of the *Plasmodium*'s life cycle, which occurs in the human host, the parasite resides for a while outside the erythrocyte; this is called the *exoerythrocytic phase*. The most effective agent for eradicating the parasite during this phase is primaquine.
7. Before administering primaquine, Professor Henson should be given a pregnancy test. This is a pregnancy category C agent, so you will need to know if certain precautions are needed in Professor Henson's case. She should also be assessed for hypersensitivity, anemia, lupus erythematosus, methemoglobinemia, porphyria, rheumatoid arthritis, methemoglobin reductase deficiency, and G6PD deficiency.
8. Mefloquine is indicated for the treatment of chloroquine-resistant malaria.
9. Each of these three patients have protozoal infections. The patient with the intestinal disorder has giardiasis. The AIDS patient has pneumocystosis, and the sexually transmitted disease is called trichomoniasis.
10. Oxamniquine increases the permeability of the worm's cell membrane to calcium, resulting in the influx of calcium ions. This causes the worms to be dislodged from their usual site in the mesenteric veins and moves them into the liver, where they are killed by host tissue reactions. Dislodgement of worms is the result of contraction and paralysis of their musculature and subsequent immobilization of their suckers, which causes the worms to detach from the blood vessel wall and be passively dislodged by normal blood flow.

CHAPTER 41
Antiseptic and Disinfectant Agents

Critical Thinking Crossword

Across
 1. Zephiran
 3. Nosocomial
 4. Aldehyde
 6. Betadine
 7. Hibiclens
 9. Dakins

Down
 2. Antiseptic
 4. Acetic
 5. Disinfectant
 8. Lysol

Multiple-choice

1. a
2. d
3. d
4. a
5. b

CHAPTER 42
Antiinflammatory, Antirheumatoid, and Related Agents

1. b
2. b
3. c
4. c
5. d
6. Symptoms of both salicylism (chronic salicylate intoxication) and acute salicylate overdose are similar except that in the acute form the effects are often more pronounced and they occur more quickly. Acute salicylate overdose results from the ingestion of a single toxic dose. Chronic salicylate intoxication occurs as a result of either high doses or prolonged therapy with high doses.
7. Acute salicylate overdose treatment consists of removing the salicylate from the GI tract and preventing its absorption; correcting fluid, electrolyte, and acid-base disturbances; and implementing measures to enhance salicylate elimination.
8. Mr. Chesney has an acute overdose of an NSAID. If it progresses, symptoms can include intense headache, dizziness, cerebral edema, cardiac arrest, and even death.
9. His treatment will consist of induced emesis by either syrup of ipecac or gastric lavage, fol-

Copyright © 2002 by Mosby, Inc. All rights reserved.

lowed by activated charcoal. Finally, supportive and symptomatic treatment will be implemented.

10. Mr. Henry needs to know that compliance with the entire medical regimen is important for the success of the treatment of gout. Allopurinol should be given with meals to try to prevent the occurrence of GI symptoms, such as nausea, vomiting, and anorexia. Fluids should be increased to 3 or 4 liters per day, and hazardous activities should be avoided if dizziness or drowsiness occurs with the medication. Also, alcohol and caffeine should be avoided since these drugs will increase uric acid levels and decrease the levels of allopurinol.

CHAPTER 43
Immunosuppressant Agents

1. b
2. c
3. c
4. a
5. d
6. a. Cyclosporine can help prevent organ rejection; if her immune system cannot recognize the new heart as foreign, it will not mount an immune response against it.
   b. Laboratory studies should include Hgb level, Hct, WBC, and platelet count. These studies should be done before, during, and after therapy; should the leukocyte count drop below $3000/mm^3$, the drug should be discontinued.
7. a. Encourage her to take it with meals or mixed with chocolate milk to prevent stomach upset.
   b. The antifungal agent is not related to her GI problems but is added several days before surgery as prophylaxis for *Candida* infections.
8. Tess is experiencing symptoms consistent with side/adverse effects of muromonab-CD3. You might suggest switching her to azathioprine, which is also used in renal transplants, but does not affect the respiratory or cardiovascular systems in the same way as her present drug.
9. First, of course, remember that Tess was switched to azathioprine in response to problems raised in question 8. More pertinent, however, is the fact that she has become an immediate candidate for transplant. Therefore, whether she has remained on muromonab-CD3 or was switched to azathioprine, she must take the drug via an oral route for several days before transplant surgery, if possible. This

avoids the risk of infection associated with injections.

CHAPTER 44
Immunizing Agents

1. a. varicella vaccine
   b. active
   c. active
   d. *H. influenzae* type b prophylaxis
   e. hepatitis B virus vaccine inactivated
   f. Rh_o (D) immune globulin
   g. passive
   h. active
   i. TB prophylaxis
   j. active
   k. diphtheria, tetanus, and pertussis prophylaxis, pediatric
   l. passive
   m. postexposure passive tetanus prophylaxis
   n. active
   o. diphtheria and tetanus prophylaxis (adult only)
2. b
3. d
4. a
5. a
6. c
7. Sometimes, after vaccination, the levels of antibodies against a particular pathogen decline over time, and a second dose of the vaccine is given to restore the antibody titers to a level that can protect the person against the infection. This second dose is referred to as a booster shot.
8. Each year a new influenza vaccine is developed that contains the three influenza virus strains that represent those strains that are likely to circulate in the United States in the upcoming winter. The vaccination from last year may not be effective for the influenza virus strains in the current year.
9. Carl may experience localized swelling, redness, discomfort, and heat at the injection site. Acetaminophen and rest are recommended for the relief of these side effects, and warm compresses on the injection site may also help to ease some of the discomfort.

CHAPTER 45
Antineoplastic Agents

Critical Thinking Crossword

Across
1. Bifunctional
6. Emetic

Copyright © 2002 by Mosby, Inc. All rights reserved.

9. Folic
11. Malignancy
12. Extravasation
13. Nadir

Down
2. Leucovorin
3. Benign
4. Leukemia
5. Spread
7. Alkylation
8. Mitosis
10. Limiting

Multiple-choice

1. d
2. c
3. c
4. b
5. a
6. a
7. b
8. d
9. a

CHAPTER 46
Biologic Response Modifiers

1. e
2. a
3. g
4. b
5. h
6. d
7. c
8. d
9. b
10. c
11. d
12. a
13. In addition to the more general assessment strategies, you should assess the patient for underlying diseases, such as cardiac conditions, and watch for contraindications, such as a hypersensitivity to proteins of *E. coli*. It is imperative that you ensure that interleukin-2 is not given with antineoplastics. Before treatment begins and then twice weekly during therapy, check the patient's serum laboratory values, such as CBC, platelet levels, BUN, creatinine, urinalysis, aspartate transaminase (AST), and alkaline phosphatase. Neutrophil counts must also be documented.
14. a. Material should reflect discussions of goals, criteria, and nursing diagnoses in the text. These are all fairly universal among the BRMs, so they will be the same for these two patients.
    b. Differences in Mr. Letti's assessment must have included the following: Contraindications he was assessed for would have included egg proteins, IgG, and neomycin. He would also be assessed for cardiac disease, angina, CHF, COPD, diabetes mellitus, bleeding disorders, bone marrow depression, and convulsive disorders. In addition, he was undoubtedly assessed for infection, CBC, level of consciousness, mental status, and confusion.
15. Sargramostim should be administered after reconstitution with 1-ml sterile water without preservatives for injection, and the vial should not be shaken. For IV infusions, dilute the medication in 0.9% NaCl. If the final concentration is less than 10 µg/ml, you should add human albumin to the NaCl to make a final concentration of 0.1% before adding the sargramostim. Give within 6 hours after reconstitution.

CHAPTER 47
Antacids and Acid Controllers

1. h
2. e
3. i
4. k
5. c
6. a
7. f
8. d
9. b
10. g
11. d
12. d
13. a
14. c
15. b
16. Side effects for omeprazole should reflect those listed in Table 47-6. However, given Mrs. Knopf's specific concerns, be sure that diarrhea, abdominal pain, vomiting, nausea, and anorexia are mentioned.
17. Patients with CHF or hypertension should use low-sodium antacids such as Riopan, Maalox, or Mylanta II. He should also be told to take the antacid without any other medications (unless specifically instructed to do so) because the antacid will interfere with the absorption of the other medications. Antacids may be taken within 1 to 2 hours after other medications. If symptoms continue or get worse, he should consult his health care provider.

Copyright © 2002 by Mosby, Inc. All rights reserved.

18. Antacids may promote premature dissolving of the enteric coating; if the coating is destroyed early in the stomach, GI upset may occur. He should take the aspirin tablets with food, not with antacids.

CHAPTER 48
Antidiarrheals and Laxatives

Critical Thinking Crossword

Across
1. Saline
4. Bulk-forming
7. Hyperosmotic

Down
2. Adsorbent
3. Anticholinergic
5. Emollient
6. Stimulant
8. Opiates

Multiple-choice and short answer

1. a
2. b
3. d
4. c
5. c
6. Darkening of the tongue and/or stool is a temporary and harmless side effect associated with bismuth subsalicylate (Pepto-Bismol).
7. The belladonna-alkaloid preparations, such as Donnatal, are contraindicated in patients with narrow-angle glaucoma.
8. a. Lactobacillus acidophilus is indicated for diarrhea caused by antibiotic treatment that has destroyed the normal intestinal flora.
   b. No! Lactobacillus normally lives in the GI tract.
9. Several factors may be causing Hillary's constipation: lack of proper exercise, poor diet (which might involve inadequate roughage and an excess of dairy products), aluminum-containing antacids, and stress.
10. a. The bulk-forming laxatives tend to produce normal stools, have few systemic effects, and are among the safest available.
    b. Ira should mix the medication with at least 6 to 8 ounces of fluid, and drink it immediately.
11. a. Because glycerin is very mild, it is often used in children.
    b. Abdominal bloating and rectal irritation.

12. a. It will probably be determined based on Kyle's weight.
    b. Contact the physician immediately.

CHAPTER 49
Antiemetic (Antinausea) Agents

1. a
2. c
3. d
4. c
5. b
6. If Norman is taking levodopa for his Parkinson's disease, the beneficial effects of the levodopa could be reduced or canceled because of a drug interaction with the neuroleptic.
7. a. Petra should take the metoclopramide 30 minutes before meals and at bedtime.
   b. Petra should be cautioned about taking her medication with alcohol because of the possible toxicity and CNS depression that can occur.
8. a. There are no significant drug interactions associated with the serotonin blockers such as ondansetron.
   b. The headache is caused by the ondansetron and can be relieved with an analgesic.
9. Thiethylperazine maleate cannot be given IV because it can cause severe hypotension. To prevent site irritation, the injection should be given deep in the upper outer quadrant of the gluteal muscle.

CHAPTER 50
Vitamins and Minerals

1. c
2. g
3. b
4. h
5. e
6. k
7. i
8. d
9. j
10. a
11. l
12. f
13. a
14. b
15. d
16. c
17. d
18. By *endogenous*, the physician was referring to the endogenous synthesis of a form of vitamin D produced in the skin by UV irradiation.

Copyright © 2002 by Mosby, Inc. All rights reserved.

Dietary sources include fish oils, salmon, sardines, and herring; fortified milk, bread, and cereals; and animal livers, tuna fish, eggs, and butter.

19. a. Broad-spectrum antibiotics can induce broad-spectrum inhibition of the intestinal flora.
    b. Vitamin K is essential for the synthesis of blood coagulation factors, which takes place in the liver.
    c. Deficiency states can also be seen in newborns because of malabsorption attributable to inadequate amounts of bile or selected drugs, and as a result of the administration of specific anticoagulants that inhibit hepatic vitamin K activity.
    d. Dietary sources of vitamin K_1 are green leafy vegetables (cabbage, spinach, etc.), meats, and milk.

20. Pernicious anemia. Ms. Evans' patient education card should focus on foods containing cyanocobalamin, which is present in foods of animal origin such as liver, kidney, fish, shellfish, meat, and dairy foods.

21. Because of venous irritation, calcium should be given via an IV infusion pump when given IV. It should be given slowly to avoid cardiac dysrhythmia and cardiac arrest. The physician, however, is correct in ordering infusion with 1% procaine. This will reduce vasospasm and dilute the effects of calcium on surrounding tissues. In either case, monitor for extravasation; if it occurs, you should discontinue administration immediately.

CHAPTER 51
Nutritional Supplements

Critical Thinking Crossword

Across
1. Erythromycin
4. Anabolism
5. Gastrostomy
8. Absorptive
10. Fatty acid
11. Essential
12. Nitrogen

Down
2. Catabolism
3. Enteral
6. Semiessential
7. Metabolism
8. Arginine
9. Phlebitis

Multiple-choice and short answer
1. a
2. c
3. b
4. c
5. a
6. d
7. a. Advantages of the newer tubes are that they are thinner and more pliable for better patient tolerance. However, they also make checking for gastric aspiration more difficult.
    b. If your attempt at gastric aspiration is unsuccessful, instill air and auscultate over the gastric area. Air sounds in the stomach denote accurate placement. Place the end of the tube in water to test for air bubbles, which signify incorrect placement.
8. Mr. Robbins shows signs of fluid overload. The first thing you should do is slow his infusion rate, then remain with him, and contact the physician immediately. Continually assess his vital signs. Next time you can prevent this by maintaining IV rates, assessing the IV infusion every hour, and monitoring the patient's fluid status.

CHAPTER 52
Blood-Forming Agents

1. a
2. b
3. c
4. d
5. a
6. Anyone who is about to receive his first dose of iron dextran is at risk for fatal anaphylaxis. Because of this, a test dose of 25 mg of iron dextran should be administered by the chosen route and appropriate method of administration. An anaphylactic reaction should occur within a few moments, although waiting at least 1 hour before giving the rest of the initial dose is recommended. IM iron should be administered deep in large muscle mass using a Z-track method and a 19- or 20-gauge, 2- to 3-inch needle.
7. Foods other than dietary sources of iron may help with iron absorption. These foods include orange juice, veal, and fish. Conversely, eggs, corn, beans, and many cereal products containing phytates may impair iron absorption. In addition, ascorbic acid enhances the absorption of iron, but antacids decrease the absorption of iron.
8. Treatment should include suction and maintenance of the airway, correction of acidosis,

Copyright © 2002 by Mosby, Inc. All rights reserved.

and control of shock and dehydration with IV fluids or blood, oxygen, and vasopressor. Abdominal radiographs can allow visualization of the tablet. A serum concentration greater than 300 µg/dl will place David at serious risk for toxicity. His stomach should be emptied immediately. Since many of the iron products are extended-release formulations that release contents in the intestines rather than in the stomach, whole gut lavage is generally believed to be superior and more effective, followed by a saline cathartic or possible surgical removal of intake iron tablets.

9. Patients with severe symptoms will exhibit coma, shock, or seizures. Chelation therapy with deferoxamine should be initiated.

CHAPTER 53
Dermatologic Agents

1. a
2. b
3. a
4. b
5. c

6. You may first ask Mr. Mugler for allergies to other forms. If he has an allergy to a particular antibacterial agent, that agent should not be used topically either. If testing for culture and sensitivity, be sure to collect the specimen before the first application of the antibacterial agent. In this case, you can simply apply a thin film of clindamycin and assess for allergy to clindamycin and other antibiotics.

7. Gloves are not only to prevent contamination from secretions, but also to prevent absorption of the medication through the skin of the person applying the medication.

8. The drug is usually applied two times a day, but the application technique will depend on the site where Ms. Goodman needs it. In any location, you will monitor Ms. Goodman's serum cortisol levels every other month if she is to receive the drug long-term. Be careful with her occlusive dressings because these can lead to follicle infections, heat retention, or systemic effects.

9. Mr. Lacroix and his children are being treated for head lice. Tell him the following: "Leave the shampoo on for 4 minutes, then rinse and dry the hair. Then use a nit comb to remove nits (eggs) from the hair shafts." Other measures he should take include decontaminating the clothing and personal articles of the infested persons. All clothing, linens, stuffed

toys, etc. should be washed in hot, soapy water, or dry-cleaned.

10. The patient taking tretinoin should avoid UV light, weather extremes, sunlight, abrasive cleansers, and other keratolytic products. Sunscreen should be worn during therapy. Tretinoin is applied to dry skin each night at bedtime, 30 minutes after cleansing. Application to wet skin may cause increased redness or drying. Benzoyl peroxide generally produces signs of improvement in 4 to 6 weeks, and side effects are infrequent and rarely a problem. Most are confined to the skin and involve peeling skin, red skin, or a sensation of warmth. Benzoyl peroxide is applied by lotion, bar, or cream sparingly.

CHAPTER 54
Ophthalmic Agents

1. c
2. h
3. j
4. k
5. a
6. d
7. b
8. f
9. g
10. e
11. c
12. b
13. b
14. d
15. a

16. The effect is less pronounced in individuals with dark eyes (brown or hazel) because pigment absorbs the drugs, and dark eyes have more pigment than light eyes (blue).

17. a. Patrice needs to demonstrate adequate knowledge of the medication and technique for administering it. She should be aware of the side effects associated with the agent (such as blurred vision, bronchospasm, nausea, vomiting, bradycardia, hypotension, and sweating); and she should know that she might experience decreased night visual acuity, stinging sensation, dull ache, or tearing on instillation. She should also be told to call the physician if these symptoms worsen.

   b. Yes. The topically applied miotic drugs can cause systemic effects; the most severe and prolonged effects are seen with the long-acting anticholinesterases (of which echothiophate is one).

Copyright © 2002 by Mosby, Inc. All rights reserved.

c. Treatment is 0.4 to 2 mg of atropine administered IM or IV. In addition, pralidoxime may be required to reverse paralysis induced by this agent.

18. a. Dipivefrin (Propine), a prodrug of epinephrine, has better lipophilicity than epinephrine and can penetrate into the anterior chamber of the eye. It is 4 to 11 times as potent as epinephrine in reducing IOP.
   b. Mrs. Ngo should report any stinging, burning, itching, lacrimation, or puffiness of the eye.
   c. No. Systemic effects are rare; they include cardiovascular effects and possibly headaches and faintness.

19. Ned may have had an allergic reaction to a preservative, such as benzalkonium chloride, in the first agent that was tried. Timolol is available in a preservative-free product.

20. a. Oral glycerin is indicated before iridectomy to reduce IOP in individuals with acute narrow-angle glaucoma. It can be flavored with lemon or lime juice and poured over cracked ice.
   b. Mrs. O'Rourke should lie flat during and after oral administration of glycerin to diminish any headache caused by cerebral dehydration.

21. a. Purulent drainage or exudate would inhibit the product's effectiveness.
   b. The solution must have been dark; in that case, it should be discarded.

22. The NSAIDs are considered less toxic, and they are preferred over the corticosteroids as initial topical therapy.

23. Stinging is normal after instillation of the drops; Ms. Luna should not wear her contact lenses while taking this medication.

CHAPTER 55
Otic Agents

1. c
2. d
3. b
4. a
5. c
6. The patient needs medical care right away; his symptoms may be indicative of head trauma.
7. To take advantage of their additional antiinflammatory, antipruritic, and antiallergic drug effects.
8. a. Clean the ear, remove all cerumen by irrigation, and clean the dropper with alcohol.
   b. The dosage is the same for adults and children: 2 to 3 drops 3 times daily.

c. He might become dizzy, so he should be supine when the drops are instilled.

9. a. The hydrocortisone will help reduce the inflammation and itching associated with the infection.
   b. A drug hypersensitivity or a perforated eardrum would be a contraindication to the use of an antibiotic or combination product containing neomycin sulfate, polymyxin B sulfate, or hydrocortisone.

10. Many ear disorders involve pain and inflammation; the anesthetic effect of the local anesthetic agents makes them beneficial in these disorders.

11. a. The instructions are different for each boy. The pinna should be held up and back during instillation of eardrops in children older than 3 years, like Drew. For children 3 years of age and younger, like Ben, the pinna should be gently pulled down and back.
   b. Reduced pain, redness, and swelling are therapeutic effects of the medication.

12. a. Esther's husband should warm up the eardrops to body temperature by holding the bottle under warm running water, not soaking it in hot water—particularly since he should be careful to not let water get into the bottle or damage the label.
   b. Esther should not sit up right away. She should lie down on the side opposite the side of the affected ear for about 5 minutes after the agent is instilled. An alternative is for her to gently insert a small cottonball into the ear canal to keep the agent there, but the cottonball should not be forced into the ear or ear canal.

OVERVIEW OF DOSAGE CALCULATIONS

Introduction

Interpreting Medication Labels

1. Generic name: rifampin
   Trade name: Rifadin
   Unit dose: 300-mg capsule
   Total in container: 30 capsules
   Route: oral
2. Generic name: loracarbef
   Trade name: Lorabid
   Unit dose: 200 mg per 5 ml
   Total in container: 75 ml (when mixed)
   Route: oral
3. Generic name: medroxyprogesterone acetate suspension
   Trade name: Depo-Provera

Copyright © 2002 by Mosby, Inc. All rights reserved.

Unit dose:	400 mg per ml
Total in container:	2.5 ml
Route:	IM use only

Section I

Basic Conversions Using Ratio and Proportion

1. 600,000 μg
2. 1,500,000 μg
3. 5 mg
4. 5000 mg
5. 2500 mg
6. 0.9 g *(Don't forget the leading zero.)*
7. 8000 g
8. 0.75 L *(Don't forget the leading zero.)*
9. 975,000 ml
10. 0.5 L *(Don't forget the leading zero.)*
11. 960 mg
12. 1.5 gr
13. 20 ml
14. 12 tsp
15. 6 tbsp
16. 90 ml
17. 0.2 oz *(Don't forget the leading zero.)*
18. 198 lb
19. 68.2 kg *(rounded to tenths)*
20. 24.2. lb

Section II

Calculating Oral Doses

1. 1 tablet
   0.5 g = 500 mg; each tablet is 500 mg; therefore 1 tablet is needed
2. 2 tablets
   0.5 mg = 500 mcg;
   250 mcg : 1 tablet :: 500 mcg : x tablet
   Proof: $250 \times 2 = 500$; $1 \times 500 = 500$
3. 0.5 tablet
   0.25 g = 250 mg;
   500 mg : 1 tablet :: 250 mg : x tablet
   Proof: $500 \times 0.5 = 250$; $1 \times 250 = 250$
4. 20 ml
   12.5 mg : 5 ml :: 50 mg : x ml
   Proof: $12.5 \times 20 = 250$; $5 \times 50 = 250$
5. 2 tablets
   600 mg = gr x; gr v : 1 tablet :: gr x : x tablet
   Proof: gr v $\times$ 2 = gr x; $1 \times$ gr x = gr x
   NOTE: With this problem, since most are more familiar with metric doses, you may convert the dose on hand, gr v, to 300 mg. Then set up your problem:
   300 mg : 1 tab :: 600 mg : x
6. 4 ml
   0.1 g = 100 mg; 125 mg : 5 ml :: 100 mg ; x ml

Proof: $125 \times 4 = 500$; $5 \times 100 = 500$
7. 3 tablets
   0.3 g = 300 mg;
   100 mg : 1 tablet :: 300 mg : x
   Proof: $100 \times 3 = 300$; $1 \times 300 = 300$
8. 22.5 ml
   20 mEq : 15 ml :: 30 mEq : x
   Proof: $20 \times 22.5 = 450$; $15 \times 30 = 450$
9. 3 capsules
   0.15 g = 150 mg;
   50 mg : 1 capsule :: 150 mg : x
   Proof: $50 \times 3 = 150$; $1 \times 150 = 150$
10. 4 tablets
    2 g = 2000 mg;
    500 mg : 1 tablet :: 2000 mg : x
    Proof: $500 \times 4 = 2000$; $1 \times 2000 = 2000$

Section III

Reconstituting Medications

1. 2 ml
   100 mg : 1 ml :: 200 mg : x
   Proof: $100 \times 2 = 200$; $1 \times 200 = 200$
2. 1.5 ml
   40 mg : 1 ml :: 60 mg : x
   Proof: $40 \times 1.5 = 60$; $1 \times 60 = 60$
3. 0.8 ml
   10,000 U : 1 ml :: 8000 U : x
   Proof: $10,000 \times 0.8 = 8000$; $1 \times 8000 = 8000$
4. 1.5 ml
   500 mg : 1 ml :: 750 mg : x
   Proof: $500 \times 1.5 = 750$; $1 \times 750 = 750$
5. 20 ml
   125 mg : 5 ml :: 500 mg : x
   Proof: $125 \times 20 = 2500$; $5 \times 500 = 2500$
6. Choose the concentration using 4.6-ml for diluent. Using the 9.6-ml diluent would necessitate giving 3 ml IM, versus the 1.5 ml using the 4.6-ml diluent.
   1.5 ml
   200,000 U : 1 ml :: 300,000 U : x ml
   Proof: $200,000 \times 1.5 = 300,000$;
   $1 \times 300,000 = 300,000$
7. 0.75 ml
   First: Convert μg to mg: 750 μg = 0.75 mg
   1:1000 indicates 1 g in 1000 ml, or 1000 mg in 1000 ml, or 1 mg/ml.
   1 mg: 1 ml :: 0.75 mg : x
   Proof: $1 \times 0.75 = 0.75$; $1 \times 0.75 = 0.75$
8. 1 ml
   NOTE: 1:5000 indicates 1 g in 5000 ml, or 1000 mg in 5000 ml, or 0.2 mg/ml.
   0.2 mg : 1 ml :: 0.2 mg : x
   Proof: $0.2 \times 1 = 0.2$; $1 \times 0.2 = 0.2$
9. 9 ml
   NOTE: 10% indicates 10 g per 100 ml, or

Copyright © 2002 by Mosby, Inc. All rights reserved.

0.1 g/ml.
Need to ensure units that are alike: 900 mg =
    0.9 g
0.1 g : 1 ml :: 0.9 g : x
Proof: 0.1 × 9 = 0.9; 1 × 0.9 = 0.9

10. 8 ml
    NOTE: 50% indicates 50 g per 100 ml,
        or 0.5 g/ml.
    0.5 g × 1 ml :: 4 g : x
    Proof: 0.5 × 8 = 4; 1 × 4 = 4

Section IV

Pediatric Calculations

1. a. 0.46 to 36.4 mg/hr
       40 lb = 18.2 kg
       Low dose: 0.025 mg/kg/hr × 18.2 kg =
       0.455, rounded to 0.46 mg/hr
       High dose: 2 mg/kg/hr × 18.2 kg =
       36.4 mg/hr
   b. Yes, the ordered dose of 1 mg/hr falls
       within the safe range for this child.
2. a. 75 to 150 mg/dose
       33 lb = 15 kg
       Low dose: 5 mg/kg/dose × 15 kg = 75
       mg/dose
       High dose: 10 mg/kg/dose × 15 kg = 150
       mg/dose
   b. 600 mg (40 mg × 15kg = 600 mg/kg/24 hr)
   c. Yes, the ordered dose of 120 mg falls
       within the safe and therapeutic range for
       this child.
3. a. 2862 to 4770 mg/24 hr
       70 lb = 31.8 kg
       Low dose: 90 mg/kg/24 hr × 31.8 kg =
       2862 mg/24 hr
       High dose: 150 mg/kg/24 hr × 31.8 kg =
       4770 mg/24 hr
   b. 954 to 1590 mg/dose
       3 doses in 24 hours; 2862 ÷ 3 = 954
       mg/dose; 4770 ÷ 3 = 1590 mg/dose
   c. No. 1.7 g = 1700 mg, which exceeds the
       safe dosage range for this drug for this
       child. (Did you remember to convert g to
       mg?)
4. a. 0.14 to 0.36 mg/day
       15 lb = 6.8 kg.
       Low dose: 0.02 mg/kg/day × 6.8 kg =
       0.136 rounded to 0.14 mg/day.
       High dose: 0.05 mg/kg/day × 6.8 kg =
       0.34 mg/day
   b. 0.07 to 0.18 mg/dose
       "bid" doses are given twice in 24 hours.
       0.14 ÷ 2 = 0.07 mg/dose; 0.36 ÷ 2 = 0.18
       mg/dose

c. Yes, 150 µg = 0.15 mg, which falls within
    the safe range of dose. (Did you remember
    to convert µg to mg?)
5. a. 15.5 to 34.1 mg/kg/dose
       34 lb = 15.5 kg.
       Low dose: 1 mg/kg/dose × 15.5 kg = 15.5
       mg/dose.
       High dose: 2.2 mg/kg/dose × 15.5 kg =
       34.1 mg/dose.
   b. Yes, the ordered dose of 30 mg is within
       the safe and therapeutic dose for this
       child.
6. a. 60.8 to 76 mcg/kg/day
       50 lb = 22.7 kg.
       Low dose: 4 mcg/kg/day × 15.2 kg = 60.8
       mcg/day.
       High dose: 5 mcg/kg/day × 15.2 kg = 76
       mcg/day.
   b. No. The ordered dose, 0.1 mg = 100 mcg,
       which exceeds the safe and therapeutic
       dose for this child. (Did you remember to
       convert mcg to mg?)

Section V

Basic Intravenous Calculations

1. Start at STEP 1. You need to calculate the
   hourly rate.
   a. 167 ml/hr
       1000 ml: 6 hr :: x : 1 hr
       (1000 × 1) = (6 × x); 1000 = 6x;
       x = 1000/6 = 166.66 (Round to nearest
       whole number.)
       Proof: 1000 × 1 = 1000; 6 × 167 = 1002
       (slight difference due to previous round-
       ing)
       (Alternate method: 1000 ml ÷ 6 hr =
       166.67 or 167 ml/hr)
   b. 42 gtt/min (Round to nearest whole num-
       ber.)
   STEP 2:
   $\dfrac{\text{drop factor}}{\text{time (min)}}$ × hourly rate = 15/60 × 167 =
   $\qquad\qquad\qquad\qquad$ 1/4 × 200 = 50

2. Start at STEP 1. You need to calculate the
   hourly rate.
   a. 200 ml/hr
       600 ml : 3 hr :: x : 1 hr
       (600 × 1) = (3 × x); 600 = 3x;
       x = 600/3 = 200
       Proof: 600 × 1 = 600; 3 × 200 = 600
       (Alternate method: 600 ml ÷ 3 hr =
       200 ml/hr)
   b. 33 gtt/min (Round to nearest whole num-
       ber.)

Copyright © 2002 by Mosby, Inc. All rights reserved.

STEP 2:
drop factor

$\dfrac{\text{time (min)}}{} \times$ hourly rate = 10/60 × 200 =
1/6 × 200 = 33.33

3. Start at STEP 1. You need to calculate the hourly rate.
  a. 83 ml/hr
    1000 ml : 12 hr :: x : 1 hr
    (1000 × 1) = (12 × x); 1000 = 12x; x =
    1000/12 = 83.33 (Round to nearest whole number.)
    Proof: 1000 × 1 = 1000; 12 × 83 = 996
    (slight difference due to previous rounding)
    (Alternate method: 1000 ml ÷ 12 hr = 83.33 or 83 ml/hr)
  b. 21 gtt/min (Round to nearest whole number.)
STEP 2:
drop factor

$\dfrac{\text{time (min)}}{} \times$ hourly rate = 15/60 × 83 =
1/4 × 83 = 20.75 (Round to nearest whole number.)

4. Start at STEP 1. You need to calculate the hourly rate.
  a. 100 ml/hr
    200 ml : 2 hr :: x : 1 hr
    (200 × 1) = (2 × x); 200 = 2x;
    x = 200/2 = 100
    Proof: 200 × 1 = 200; 2 × 100 = 200
    (Alternate method: 200 ml ÷ 2 hr = 100 ml/hr)
  b. 100 gtt/min
STEP 2:
drop factor

$\dfrac{\text{time (min)}}{} \times$ hourly rate = 60/60 × 100 =
1 × 100 = 100
  c. The drop factor for microdrip tubing is 60 gtt/ml.

5. Start at STEP 2. The hourly rate has been provided (75 ml/hr).
  13 gtt/min (Round to nearest whole number.)
STEP 2:
drop factor

$\dfrac{\text{time (min)}}{} \times$ hourly rate = 10/60 × 75 =
1/6 × 75 = 12.5

6. Start at STEP 2. The hourly rate has been provided (75 ml/hr).
  19 gtt/min (Round to nearest whole number.)
STEP 2:
drop factor

$\dfrac{\text{time (min)}}{} \times$ hourly rate = 15/60 × 75 =
1/4 × 75 = 18.75

7. Start at STEP 2. The hourly rate has been provided (75 ml/hr).
  25 gtt/min
STEP 2:
drop factor

$\dfrac{\text{time (min)}}{} \times$ hourly rate = 20/60 × 75 =
1/3 × 75 = 25

8. As the drop factor increases, the gtt/min also increases.

9. a. 100 ml/hr
  b. and c. Since the infusion pump delivers in ml/hr, it is unnecessary to calculate gtt/min.
  Start at STEP 1. You need to calculate the hourly rate. Remember, 30 min = 0.5 hr.
  50 ml : 0.5 hr :: x ml : 1 hr
  (50 × 1) = (0.5 × x); 50 = 0.5x;
  x = 50/0.5 = 100
  Proof: 50 × 1 = 50; 0.5 × 100 = 50
  (Alternate method: 50 ml ÷ 0.5 hr = 100 ml/hr)

10. Start at STEP 1. You need to calculate the hourly rate.
  a. 125 ml/hr
    500 ml : 4 hr :: x : 1 hr
    (500 × 1) = (4 × x); 500 = 4x;
    x = 500/4 = 125
    Proof: 500 × 1 = 500; 4 × 125 = 500
    (Alternate method: 500 ml ÷ 4 hr = 125 ml/hr)
  b. 125 gtt/min
STEP 2:
drop factor

$\dfrac{\text{time (min)}}{} \times$ hourly rate = 60/60 × 125 =
1 × 125 = 125

PRACTICE QUIZ

1. 0.75 mg
  1000 μg : 1 mg :: 750 μg : x mg
  Proof: 1000 × 0.75 = 750; 1 × 750 = 750
2. 8000 mg
  1 g : 1000 mg :: 8 g : x mg
  Proof: 1 × 8000 = 8000; 1000 × 8 = 8000
3. 113.6 kg
  1 kg : 2.2 lb :: x kg : 250 lb
  Proof: 1 × 250 = 250; 2.2 × 113.6 = 249.92
  (rounds to 250)
4. 165 lb
  1 kg : 2.2 lb :: 75 kg : x lb
  Proof: 1 × 165 = 165; 2.2 × 75 = 165
5. 15 ml
  1 tsp : 5 ml :: 3 tsp : x ml
  Proof: 1 × 15 = 15; 5 × 3 = 15

Copyright © 2002 by Mosby, Inc. All rights reserved.

6. 600 mg
   gr i (1) : 60 mg :: gr x (10) : x mg
   Proof: 1 (gr i) × 600 = 600; 60 × 10 (gr x) = 600
7. 2 ml
   25 mg : 1 ml :: 50 mg : x ml
   Proof: 25 × 2 = 50; 1 × 50 = 50
8. 1 tablet
   STEP 1: Convert g to mg: 0.5 g = 500 mg
   500 mg : 1 tablet :: 500 mg: x tablet
   Proof: 500 × 1 = 500; 1 × 500 = 500
9. 2 ml
   50 mg : 1 ml :: 100 mg : x ml
   Proof: 50 × 2 = 100; 1 × 100 = 100
10. 5 ml
    1% indicates 1 g in 100 ml, which equals 1000 mg/100 ml, or 10 mg/1 ml.
    10 mg : 1 ml :: 50 mg : x ml
    Proof: 10 × 5 = 50; 1 × 50 = 50
11. 0.25 ml
    1:1000 indicates 1 g in 1000 ml, which equals 1000mg/1000 ml, or 1 mg/ml.
    1 mg : 1 ml :: 0.25 mg : x ml
    Proof: 1 × 0.25 = 0.25; 1 × 0.25 = 0.25
12. 1.5 ml
    10,000 U : 1 ml :: 15,000 U : x ml
    Proof: 10,000 × 1.5 = 15,000; 1 × 15,000 = 15,000
13. a. 0.2 to 0.8 mg/dose
    b. No, the dose of 1 mg exceeds the safe and therapeutic range for this child.
       22 lb = 10 kg
       Low range: 0.02 mg/kg/dose × 10 kg = 0.2 mg/dose
       High range: 0.08 mg/kg/dose × 10 kg = 0.8 mg/dose
14. a. 63 ml/hr
       500 ml ÷ 8 hr = 62.5, rounded to 63 ml/hr
    b. 16 gtt/min
       $\dfrac{\text{drop factor}}{\text{time (min)}}$ × hourly rate = 15/60 × 63 = 1/4 × 63 = 15.75, rounded to 16 gtt/min

15. a. Infusion pumps deliver ml/hr.
    b. 50 ml/hr (as stated in the question)
16. a. 42 ml/hr
       1000 ml ÷ 24 hr = 41.67, rounded to 42 ml/hr
    b. 42 gtt/min (Remember, if the drop factor is 60, the rate is the same as the gtt/min.)
       $\dfrac{\text{drop factor}}{\text{time (min)}}$ × hourly rate = 60/60 × 42 = 1 × 42 = 42 gtt/min
17. a. 1 g
    b. 2.5 ml
    200 mg : 1 ml :: 500 mg : x ml
    Proof: 200 × 2.5 = 500; 1 × 500 = 500
18. a. 200,000 U/ml
    b. 23 ml
    c. 1 ml (concentration is 200,000 U per 1 ml)
    d. Label the multidose vial with the date, time, amount of diluent used, and user's initials.
19. a. 6 ml
       100 mg : 1 ml :: 600 mg : x ml
       Proof: 100 × 6 = 600; 1 × 600 = 600
    b. Up to 1410 mg/24 hr
       31 lb = 14.1 kg; 14.1 kg × 100 mg/kg/day = 1410 mg/24 hr (safe dose)
    c. 705 mg/dose
       There are two doses per day; 1410 mg ÷ 2 = 705 mg/dose
    d. Yes
       The ordered dose of 600 mg does not exceed the 705 maximum dose.
20. 2.5 ml
    125 μg = 0.125 mg
    0.05 mg : 1 ml :: 0.125 mg : x mg
    Proof: 0.05 × 2.5 = 0.125; 1 × 0.125 = 0.125

Copyright © 2002 by Mosby, Inc. All rights reserved.